WHOA DUDE!

Think on these things before getting too deep into smoking Weed*

*or what the science of marijuana is telling us about the harmful effects of marijuana for you, your friends or your kids.

Kevin G. Becker Ph.D.

Publisher's Cataloging-in-Publication data
Names: Becker, Kevin G., author.
Title: Whoa dude ! Think on these things before getting too deep into smoking weed : or what the science of marijuana is telling us about the harmful effects for you , your friends , or your kids / Kevin G. Becker Ph.D.
Description: Includes bibliographical references. | Baltimore, MD: Kevin G. Becker, 2021.
Identifiers: LCCN: 2021904477 | ISBN: 978-1-7367521-0-4 (paperback) | 978-1-7367521-1-1 (ebook)
Subjects: LCSH Marijuana. | Marijuana---Physiological effect. | Marijuana--Psychological aspects. | Marijuana abuse. | Cannabis. | Cannabis abuse. | Dependency (Psychology) | BISAC HEALTH & FITNESS / Cannabis & CBD | MEDICAL / Mental Health | PSYCHOLOGY / Psychopathology / Addiction | SCIENCE / Life Sciences / Neuroscience
Classification: LCC BF209.C3 .B43 2021 | DDC 616.86/35--dc23

Information in this publication is for educational and scientific purposes only and is not intended as a substitute for the advice of medical and health care professionals. The views and opinions presented here are wholly the work of Kevin G. Becker Ph.D and do not represent the views or an endorsement from the National Institutes of Health.

I have used the terms Weed, Marijuana, and Cannabis rather loosely and inter-changeably in this book. That may not be technically accurate with regard to specific scientific publications.

Contents

Chapter 3

Chapter 4

Chapter 5
Biological, Biochemical, and Genetic Basics 48

Chapter 6
Brain Stuff

Chapter 7
Cannabis and the Risk of Mental Illness

Chapter 8

Pregnancy, Neonatal Issues, and Childhood 89

Chapter 9

Other Very Important Heath-related Stuff 99

Chapter 10

List of Figures

Preface

There is a fire raging across America and around the world. It is an unstoppable grass fire; the legalization of recreational marijuana. As of this writing, it seems inevitable that cannabis legalization will happen in many states and in many countries. The flames are driven by the failed war on drugs, the desire to remedy decades of unfair marijuana related incarceration, a growing medical marijuana industry, and by the enormous profits to be made in the recreational marijuana market. Clouded by all the smoke and noise is the clear scientific evidence that long term use of marijuana and cannabis products can be harmful to the health and well being of many individuals, especially adolescents and young adults.

My motivation for writing this book is first as a brother and father and second as a scientist. I have seen the effects of weed on my immediate and extended family and friends. As a scientist, it is strangely discordant that the public, legislative, and individual belief that marijuana is safe flies in the face of a great deal of scientific evidence that marijuana can cause significant harm to your health and in your life. I hope you will learn some things. I know I did. I hope it will light a small fire in you as you think about it, discuss these issues among friends and family, and decide your own path forward.

Acknowledgments

First and foremost, I would like to thank my wife Bonnie for her support and patience in general and through the process of writing this book. I would also like to thank my sons Henry and Will for their interesting life experiences and conversations on the topic.

Special thanks to Katherine Peterson Ph.D. of the National Eye Institute, Marquis Vawter Ph.D. of the University of California at Irvine, Tanya Barrett Ph.D. of the National Center for Biotechnology Information, Philip Lee Ph.D. of the National Institute on Child Health and Human Development, Bronwen Martin Ph.D. of the University of Antwerp, and Stuart Maudsley Ph.D of the University of Antwerp for their helpful and insightful reviews and comments. I would also like to thank Marco Balpiero, Inez Thompson, Henry Gruber and Michael Gilliom for their years of kindness and support for my brother.

For all the Marks in the world,
and for all their families

Chapter 1
Introduction

Who Is This Book For?

This book is for you. If you smoke weed or use cannabis products. You are going to spend a lot of money and time with weed; shouldn't you know more about it? What it could be doing to your health?

It is for you if you are young, your friends are smoking weed, and you have questions about the health risks of weed. Is it safe? How much is too much? What are the long term effects?

It is also for you, if you are a parent, brother, sister, or a friend of someone who uses weed and are concerned about their welfare.

It is for you if you are just curious and wish to get a direct line to the scientific basis of one of the major controversies of our time.

What Is This Book About (and Not About)?

The main goal of this book is to take on two common opinions in the public sphere that are just not true. The first is, "weed never hurt anybody," and the second is, "we don't really know, there aren't a lot of scientific studies on the effects of weed." Well, there is an overwhelming amount of published peer-reviewed scientific evidence that weed causes harm in some people—not everybody—and that it has the potential to affect your health and well being. Science is a journey, there is always more to be uncovered. But, if you think there is not a lot of science about the health risks of weed...here's your chance to learn more.

This is a sourcebook about marijuana. The focus is on science, in particular, the many scientific studies on the harm that using marijuana may cause you and your friends. And for you to really understand, and delve deeper into why weed may be harmful, there is a reference section at the end of the book. That section contains the papers I have used to prepare this book. And I want you to be able to read these papers too.

When you visit the companion website, **Whoa Dude References**, found at https://whoadude-the-book.com/references/ you will be able to download and read many of the scientific papers mentioned throughout this book.

What good is it to you if I cite a reference to a scientific publication in the prestigious "*Journal of Blah Blah Blah*," but you don't have access to that publication? Not much help at all. I don't want you take my word for it. You're smart; I believe in you. So, I've made the papers easily available for you to look at. You can read a few scientific papers. You may find them interesting. You may be convinced to learn more. You might even do a little better at trivia night down at the pub on Tuesday nights.

This book is not about the potential benefits of medical marijuana and cannabidiol (CBD). Medical marijuana may hold promise for certain conditions and diseases, but much work needs to be done with regard to its safety and efficacy. Information about medical marijuana and CBD is available from your doctor.

This book is about the *recreational* use of weed in adolescents, young adults and older people. It is about the *dark side* of weed. It is a cautionary tale. And like all cautionary tales, it's about what *could* happen, not what *will* happen. In scientific parlance that is known as probability. Everything in life has a certain chance of happening and a certain chance of not happening, influenced by what you do or do not do.

There be wolves. The big bad wolf may not eat you, but you don't want to be Little Red Riding Hood skipping merrily down the lane, totally clueless to wolves behind trees. Weed may not harm *you*, but it might hurt your brother, your kid, your best friend, or that shy teenager that lives in the house three doors down. If you are into or are getting into weed, you should understand the health risks.

As more and more localities, states, and federal governments debate the legalization of medical and recreational marijuana, many people have questions about its short and long-term health effects. There is growing evidence that because weed is being legalized, people think that marijuana is safe for everyone. *This is simply not true.* If you only get your information from the internet, you are getting a mashup of myths, facts, self promotion, confirmation bias, opinion, and marketing based on greed. I have different motives in this book. I want to help you go directly to the sources of scientific information about the harmful health effects of marijuana. If you are going to spend the next 20 years smoking weed and spending a lot of cash as well...maybe put a little time getting up to speed, thinking about what this habit could possibly do to you.

This book is a discussion about the scientific evidence that marijuana can cause harm in people. This is true for people at any age, but I am emphasizing its effects on teens and young adults. We are going to look at the growing scientific evidence of marijuana and harm. This science is not finished; it is in progress, and some studies conflict or are controversial. Some evidence is strong and the connections are pretty clear, while other studies are more preliminary. But in each case, there is enough data for medical professionals to emphasize caution and concern. Let's consider what they are concerned about. There is increasing evidence to say., *Whoa Dude, let me think about this, maybe tap the brakes a bit.*

In this book, you're not going to read crazy talk like whats in "Reefer Madness" or anything simplistic like, "Just say No." These approaches are outdated and superficial in an era of marijuana decriminalization, medical marijuana dispensaries, and the legalization movement.

I personally believe in marijuana decriminalization and medicalization. The "War on Drugs" has been a colossal failure and has ruined many lives, especially in minority communities. However, I do not support the rapid aggressive commercialization of marijuana, the "Budweiser-ization" of weed, which is driven by greed and self interest; not by health concerns and science.

In today's world, you have to decide for yourself if you smoke or use weed, or not. There is so much misinformation and self promotion on the internet, its crazy. To make good decisions, you need to be well informed. When it comes to weed, like for many other things, know as much as you can about what you put in your body.

Chapter 2

Getting Your Bearings

Different Levels of Scientific Evidence; Statistical Associations versus Causality; Multiple Studies from Different Research Groups; Older Data or Newer Data In the World of Weed; PubMed and PubMed Central; Ten Excellent Free Reviews.

This book is full of honest discussions on topics of great concern to people who rigorously and independently study the effects of marijuana on the human body and its effects on society. They publish the results of these studies in peer-reviewed scientific journals. This is the gold standard of scientific analysis. In this book, you will not read opinions that are just found on the web.

What kind of studies are we going to talk about? Many kinds: cell culture studies, molecular, genetic, and statistical studies, human and animal studies, studies from different countries, population studies, meta-analyses, narrative reviews and systematic reviews. Case studies are anecdotal individual stories and are quite different than large population statistical based studies. We will discuss small studies, large studies, exploratory studies, conflicting data, confirmatory data. Each type of scientific study has its strengths and limitations. Some countries have excellent health data systems such as the U.K., Sweden or Israel, or longer experience with medical or recreational marijuana, like The Netherlands, Canada and Uruguay. Each type of study plays an important role, each has limitations.

Research into the effects of marijuana is *not* a conspiracy by big pharma. The vast majority of research described in this book is performed at universities or government research labs, and is funded primarily by government agencies like the National Institutes of Health or non-profit medical funding organizations like the Howard Hughes Medical Institute (HHMI) in the U.S. or the Wellcome Trust in the U.K. Most of the day to day research work is done by smart, hardworking, but underpaid graduate students and post-doctoral fellows. They deserve a lot of credit.

There are certain kinds of studies you can only do in animals, such as drug intervention studies in a rat brain. Besides the ethical issues of injecting experimental drugs into people, it is often very difficult to disentangle all the factors in human studies, like other underlying health conditions, socioeconomic status, genetic background, study completion, sources and potency of the weed used, and other substance use, such as alcohol and nicotine. Highly controlled, standardized testing of cannabinoids in the rat complements human studies and has been essential in teasing apart the complex effects of weed on neurobiology and behavior. I understand if you have concerns about the ethical treatment of animals in scientific studies; many people do. I share those concerns, but as a scientist, I have seen the irreplaceable value in thoughtfully using animals in research. This research improves health and saves lives.

We learn something from each type of study; it's all good. Each study increases our knowledge about the effects marijuana has on your health, your behavior, and on society. In this book, every topic will be extensively referenced. From the book's website, you can find links to these publications, so you can read the original research. My promise to you is I will give you the facts based on the research. No opinions (except where stated), no proselytizing, no diatribes about what you should or should not do. You decide. Look at the studies described in the book, read them, talk to your friends, your siblings, your parents, or a teacher. Start a rousing discussion. And then make wise informed decisions.

There Are Different Levels of Scientific Evidence

I am going to define three levels of scientific evidence that we find in scientific publications. These three levels reflect the amount of evidence amassed and the degree of certainty about a hypothesis or question. It is an acknowledgment that the scientific process is a journey. Ideas are proposed, tested, and expanded upon. Sometimes an idea falls flat and is abandoned. Sometimes a hypothesis is confirmed, and that leads to other theories and concepts. Scientific techniques, equipment, and algorithms get better over time. Science is a process.

Strong evidence

Strong evidence means that multiple independent research groups find statistically significant evidence supporting the same or similar conclusions on a topic. Characteristics of studies that contribute to this strength rating are reports that include a large number of participants, and ones that come from different countries and populations, and therefore local or regional peculiarities may be diluted. Strong evidence tends to be supported by different types of studies such as; case studies, molecular studies, small focused studies (~20 people), large population studies (>20,000 people), database comparisons, meta-analyses, animal studies, interventional studies, and other types of studies that complement and tend to support the overall concepts. This rating doesn't have to include all these kinds of studies, its just that more supporting evidence is better. There may be some conflicting or negative studies here, but the large majority of studies support the basic observations. An example of a topic with strong supporting evidence is cannabis and psychosis (see Chapter 7).

Emerging evidence

Emerging evidence is based on multiple preliminary studies in which there is an increasing amount of evidence that supports a given conclusion. Usually this includes increasingly diverse and larger studies on a specific topic. The concept doesn't have to have super strong support yet, but there is enough evidence to allow a reasonable person to say "there is something going on here." An example of a topic in which there is emerging evidence is cannabis and myocardial infarction (heart attack; see Chapter 9).

Preliminary evidence

This strength rating comes when there are a few publications making conclusions that are very interesting and may introduce new topics. All big ideas start with an initial paper. Sometimes a big claim might be made about a result, but it may not pan out upon further research, or it may grow in strength with further confirmatory studies. These are things to watch. There may be conflicting evidence as well. There might be studies that find no support or directly conflict with other studies about that topic. For example: Cannabis and Anxiety (see Chapter 7).

When can we say that something is proven? Most scientists don't use the word proof, except maybe mathematicians. The word proof is used by the general public. Most scientists constantly weigh the evidence for a hypothesis. When the evidence becomes strong or convincing, then the hypothesis becomes generally accepted as correct. But that consensus can change if new, contrary evidence comes to light. Science makes room for conflicting evidence. That's how science works: different research groups amassing evidence; different hypotheses duking it out.

Sometimes people don't accept a finding until causality is strictly shown, even when there is a great deal of supporting evidence. You can often make wise personal health decisions when evidence is still emerging and is becoming clearer, rather than waiting until formal causality is proven, which may be a long time in coming, if ever. It was generally accepted by the public that cigarette smoking caused lung cancer, while industry spokesman denied that finding. (Sometimes, causality is viewed in the rear view mirror, only after great harm has occurred.)

Statistical Associations versus Causality

An important distinction in science is between a statistical association and direct causality. An association is when one thing is very often found with a condition. Many times the association is identified by various mathematically rigorous statistical tests. Causality is when a condition is directly caused by that thing. Establishing causality is not simple to do. Quite often an association is due to direct causality, but other times things are tangled and complex. There are times when you can only identify a statistical association, and you personally are certain that it is real, but as hard as you try, you can't figure out the cause (science never cuts you a break).

Sometimes an effect is caused by many inputs, not just by A, it can be A + B with a C kicker. And sometimes an association can be purely coincidental. There is probably a high statistical correlation between Seattle grunge rock and the increasing use of cell phones. They both took off in the mid 1980s into the early 1990s; purely coincidental.

Many statistical associations are rock solid and hold up, but sometimes associations are spurious and fall apart. Quite often statistical associations are identified in large population studies. Scientists may then try to establish direct causality through focused molecular or animal studies.

Why Multiple Studies from Different Research Groups Strengthen a Scientific Finding

If a particular scientific conclusion comes just from one research group, be skeptical, the jury is still out on whether it's real or not. That's why a splashy new report in the media of a novel finding is suspect until it is confirmed independently. If different independent groups, from different universities, come to the same conclusion, that strengthens the hypothesis. If different types of studies, such as population statistical studies, molecular studies, and animal studies, all support that hypothesis, that's even better. If a hypothesis is tested by different groups in different countries, even better. So if you see that a health risk from cannabis is found in the United States, Australia, Sweden, Brazil, and Canada, that's super strong evidence.

Why It Matters Whether We Look at Older Data or Newer Data In the World of Weed

If human population studies of cannabis use older data collected by self reporting or personal use, those studies may not reflect the much higher potency of weed today or of increasing cannabis availability due to legalization. Some studies by design include older data. For example, longitudinal studies which look at populations over many years are well established and important types of studies. However, one potential downside to a longitudinal study about marijuana is that the longer it looks back in time, the more likely the study will be confounded by the very different potencies of weed and weed extracts then and now, and the greater access to marijuana currently. Sometimes, authors note these differences and correct for them statistically. A meta-analysis or a systematic analysis is a report that aggregates many different studies on a topic. These may include older studies, but may not account for the higher THC concentrations or greater access to weed today. When you are reading a study that includes older data on weed from human studies, such as ones that use self-reporting or questionnaires, look to see if the authors have accounted for the differences in potency and availability over time.

How to get and read scientific and medical papers directly from PubMed (sometimes free) or PubMed Central (always free)

When it comes to informing the public, one of the main problems with scientific publishing is that quite often it is just *scientists talking to scientists*. Many times important information doesn't get out into the general public or is forgotten after today's news cycle. Another huge issue which feeds into that, is that in many cases you may have to pay for access to scientific papers. However, more and more, with open access scientific publishing, reading scientific and medical publications is free. I will highlight those papers that are free and you can download and read them directly.

I encourage you to try to read the scientific papers discussed here. This is important stuff. Download them, send them to other interested people. Send them to people who are not so interested. Present them as reports in science or health class. Give them to your kids. Explain them to your grandmother.

Here is a trick to reading scientific papers for the novice. Don't read them in order. Read the Title and Abstract first, then the Conclusion, then the Introduction, then the Discussion. If you are still hanging in there, get into the Results, then the Methods. Don't get discouraged if you don't understand all the details. Quite often a novice will blast through a paper and get bogged down in the methods and specific detailed results and cry out

"I don't understand!!" Try to get an overall impression of the paper before you get up to your eyeballs in the specific details.

Another hint is that every scientific paper has the email address of the communicating author, usually in the affiliations on the Abstract or first page. Email them, ask them questions. Quite often they will send you a copy of the article. Keep the discussion going. Invite them to give a talk; they love that.

PubMed is the main public website where you can search directly for scientific and biomedical published papers. It contains over 30 million citations for biomedical literature from the MEDLINE database, hosted by the National Center for Biotechnology Information at the U.S. National Institutes of Health. It is an enormously valuable resource for you, important in your health, for medical information and scientific discovery.

The easiest way to search PubMed for the papers referenced here is with the PubMed ID number (PMID). Each scientific reference in this book has a PMID number, (and/or PubMed Central ID) at the end of the reference. Go to the PubMed website: https://www.ncbi.nlm.nih.gov/pubmed and type just the number in the PubMed search box and hit enter. What you will see is the Title and Abstract for that paper. In the upper right corner you may find Full Text Links. Click on any of those to go directly to read the paper. Sometimes the journals website is open access and free, but sometimes there is a charge. Sometimes there is no link to the paper.

You may see references with a PMC number and a link to PubMed Central (PMC). https://www.ncbi.nlm.nih.gov/pmc/

PubMed Central, is the repository of free open access subset of PubMed, directly linked to the paper. It is newer, smaller in scope, and complimentary to PubMed. I encourage you to go right to the papers, read them yourself. Download them and send them to other folks. If a reference in this book has a PMC number, you can go directly to the free PubMed Central website and enter the PMC number in the search box to get direct access to the paper. I will highlight the reference if there is a free source for that particular reference.

Also check out the Whoa Dude free website where you will find a list of all the references in the book. You can click through directly to many of the abstracts, papers or websites referenced. Whoa Dude Online References https://whoadude-the-book.com/references

Ten Excellent Free Reviews for You to Read On the Possible health Effects of Weed

A scientific review paper is a broad look at a topic by experts who have worked in a field for a long time. Reviews contain a thoughtful discussion with many citations to support the discussion. Here are ten excellent free reviews on the harmful effects of weed, I am putting them right here, rather than burying them in the references because its important, take a look at some or all of them. Your homework is to read at least one, there is no test. I have read almost certainly over 10,000 scientific papers in my life, I'm just asking you to read at least one. Any one of these review papers will get you up to speed. Read all ten and you will be the expert.

Go to PubMedCentral https://www.ncbi.nlm.nih.gov/pmc/ and search with the PMC number found after each reference.

1. Macdonald K. and Pappas K.. WHY NOT POT? A Review of the Brain based Risks of Cannabis. Innovations in Clinical Neuroscience 2016;13{3-4}:13-22. PubMed PMID_27354924_ PubMed Central PMC4911936.[1]

2. Volkow, N. et. al. Adverse Health Effects of Marijuana Use. New England Journal of Medicine. 2014 Jun 5; 370{23}: 2219–2227. PubMed PMID24897085_PubMed Central PMC4827335.[2]

3. Zehra A. et al. 2018 Cannabis Addiction and the Brain: a Review Journal of Neuroimmune Pharmacology 2018; 13{4}: 438–452. PubMed PMID29556883_PubMed Central PMC6223748.[3]

4. Memedovich KA, et al. The adverse health effects and harms related to marijuana use: an overview review CMAJ Open 2018. PubMed PMID30115639_PubMed Central PMC6182105.[4]

5. Murray, R.M. et al. Traditional marijuana, high-potency cannabis and synthetic cannabinoids: increasing risk for psychosis World Psychiatry. 2016 Oct; 15{3}: 195–204. PubMed PMID27717258_ PubMed Central PMC5032490.[5]

6. Grant C and Belanger . Cannabis and Canada's Children and Youth. Paediatr Child Health 2017 May;22{2}:98-102. PubMed PMID29480902_ PubMed Central PMC5804770.[6]

7. De Aquino JP, Sherif M, Radhakrishnan R, Cahill JD, Ranganathan M, D'Souza DC. The Psychiatric Consequences of Cannabinoids. Clin Ther. 2018 Sep;40{9}:1448-1456 PubMed PMID29678279.[7]

8. Hasin DS US Epidemiology of Cannabis Use and Associated Problems. Neuropsychopharmacology. 2018 Jan; 43{1}: 195–212. PubMed PMID28853439_PubMed Central PMC5719106.[8]

9. Archie S.R. and Cucullo L. Front Pharmacol. Harmful Effects of Smoking Cannabis: A Cerebrovascular and Neurological Perspective. 2019; 10: 1481. PubMed PMID31920665_ PubMed Central PMC6915047.[9]

10. Beverly HK, Castro Y, Opara I. Age of First Marijuana Use and Its Impact on Education Attainment and Employment Status. J Drug Issues. PubMed PMID31341332_PubMed Central PMC6655417.[10]

Chapter 3

Things to know about Weed

The Big 4-How early, How often, How much, How strong; Low Dose/High Dose–Short Term/Long Term use; People are different; This is not the marijuana of the 1969 Woodstock generation;

To jump into the science of the harmful effects of marijuana you first have to become familiar with some important concepts in relation to weed.

1. *The first set of important things to think about is what I call:* The *BIG FOUR*. *They are:*

- how early
- how often
- how much, and
- how strong

The age you start using weed, how often you use it, how much you consume, and its potency are all directly related to the potential for bad outcomes in almost *everything* described in this book.

As you will read later on, marijuana can affect many complex processes including brain function and development, motivation, and your emotional state. The age you start using weed is especially important in how it could alter those critical stages of development and affect your life through the teen years and into adulthood. A national survey in the United States of almost 45,000 teenagers from 1975 to 2015 reported that 12% of 8th graders (ages 13-14), 25% of 10th graders (ages 15-16) and 35% of 12th graders (ages 17-18) have used marijuana in the past year[11].

Beginning marijuana use in the early teen years has been shown to increase the chance of symptoms of drug abuse later in life. A study of cannabis use in 1,030 boys ages 13-17 reported that those who started using cannabis before age 15 were at a higher risk of developing drug abuse symptoms by age 28. They further state that, "the odds of developing any drug abuse symptoms by 28 were reduced by 31% for each year of delayed cannabis use onset[12]."

The age when you start smoking weed can also have an impact on your education and future employment(see Chapter 10). A study from the University of Texas showed that those who reported first using marijuana between the ages of 12 and 14 had a less chance of completing high school than those that started between the ages of 15 and 17[10].

Early marijuana use can also influence the age at which you may get psychological problems, including psychosis, depression and anxiety. A study from Harvard Medical School demonstrated that that the age at onset of cannabis was directly associated with age at onset of psychosis[13]. A comprehensive review of the scientific literature in 2019 stressed the importance of the age of first marijuana use on psychosis, depression and anxiety in those under the age of 25[14]. The title of a recent scientific paper from the University of Miami spells it out, "Smoking Cannabis and Acquired Impairments in Cognition: Starting Early Seems Like a Really Bad Idea"[15].

How often you use weed and how much you use at any age are both central to the discussion of marijuana related harm to your health. In some ways it's similar with cigarettes, alcohol, ice cream, and many other things in life. Having a bowl of ice cream is not going to make you fat. Eating a big bowl of ice cream three times a week for thirty years may lead to obesity, diabetes, and heart disease. Smoking a joint at a party is not going to kill you. Beginning to use weed at age 14 and then using it often through your teen years when your brain development is in full swing; that's risky behavior[16]. Doing the "wake and bake"[17] or smoking weed nearly every day, just to take the edge off can lead to dependence, addiction, increasing anxiety, depression, and other health complications. At some point you may cross a line, and while that line is different for different people, these are bad health outcomes. Consider whether you want to put yourself at risk.

Figure 1. How frequently you smoke or use weed.

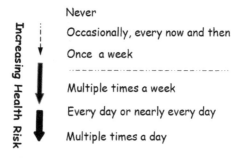

In addition to how often and how much you use, the health risks also increase with increasingly stronger cannabis and cannabis products. The effects of potency goes for cannabis products as well, eating THC edibles with 50% THC, then saying "dude, do you feel anything, I don't feel anything"...and eating more[18], could send you straight to the emergency ward[18-20].

2. *The second important concept is*: Low Dose/High Dose and Short Term/Long Term use.

There is a sweet spot in spices; salt, pepper, sugar, medicines and many other things we take into our bodies. Low dose and/or short term use-not so bad; High dose and/or long term use-bad. These effects are related to the concept of Dose-Response.

There are many examples in this book where cannabis may have a "bi-phasic effect"[21, 22]. Short term use, also referred to as acute use, or a low dose of weed in some cases, not all, may not be harmful or maybe even beneficial, but long term use, also referred to as chronic, daily or near daily use, or higher potency weed, may have increasingly cumulative harmful effects. Studies in animals also support this low dose ok-high dose bad concept. This is true in many things in life as well.

Let me stress that although there are examples of low dose-ok: high dose-bad with cannabis use, there is emerging evidence that even low doses or a single use of cannabis can cause harm[23], including psychosis[24]. It is reflective of the complex-ity of neurobiological responses and individual differences in response to cannabis.

What is a Dose-Response Relationship and why is it important?

With many drugs, both medicinal drugs and drugs of abuse, there is an effective range where the drug works; too little is not effective, too much can cause harm or even death. This is called a Dose-Response Relation-ship[25]. For example, certain cancer drugs work only in a specific range, too little doesn't work; too much can kill you. If you read a scientific study of Cannabis and they demonstrate a dose-response relationship; that bad health outcomes appear with an increasing dose or potency, that is a good indication that that scientific result is true. For example, epidemiological data for Cannabis use shows a Dose-Response Relationship with psychosis outcomes[26]. It should be clearly noted that there are studies that show "single doses of cannabis and THC cause a dose dependent reduction in performance as assessed with neurocognitive tasks measuring memory, attention, impulse control and motor function"[27-32].

3. The third important concept is: People are different.
Different people respond differently to things that affect their health. In scientific circles this is known as clinical heterogeneity. We all know people who are skinny, can eat anything and as much as they want, and they don't get fat. But for other people its, "once on the lips, forever on the hips". For them, eating and weight can be a constant struggle. The reasons for this are a complex mashup of behavior, genetics, impulsivity, social cues, family history, your particular metabolism and many other factors. It is similar for response to weed. A recent striking example of individual health variation is the COVID-19 crisis. About 25-80% of people who were exposed to the virus were asymptomatic, many didn't even know they were infected. Some people who got sick just had flu like symptoms, while others had a high fever, chills, muscle aches and coughing, ~5% were hospitalized, and ~1-3% died[33]. Same virus... different people, different health outcomes. Just as important is that different health outcomes can occur at different ages and with different underlying conditions. People are different.

We now live in the world of "personalized medicine" where each person is seen as a unique individual with personal strengths and risks. What may be ok for you with weed might not be ok for your friend, your neighbor, or somebody with a family history of mental illness or substance abuse. Your individual risk profile contributes to whether or not you or the people around you could be at risk for health problems associated with weed.

Most people who drink alcohol do not become alcoholics. Most people who ever smoke cigarettes do not get lung cancer, and most people who ever smoke weed don't experience paranoia and psychosis[34] or other serious complications, but...(wait for it)...*some do*. When they do, it can be devastating and life changing. My guess is you probably don't want to be that person. Nobody wants to be a statistic.

The majority of people don't have bad outcomes from any single bad thing.

Just because *you* may not have a bad outcome due to weed doesn't mean other people might not. If you read cannabis blogs and forums on the internet, they are filled with longtime users saying, "I've been smoking weed for 40 years, and I have never had a problem." Good for them, they dodged the bullet...they are lucky.

Different people have their own complex health resiliency and vulnerabilities, only a subset of people may get affected. This is how many afflictions work. This is where probability comes in. Most people don't get appendicitis; but ~7% do. Most women don't get breast cancer; but ~13% do. Most people don't get Parkinson's disease; but ~1% do. If you have not gotten any of these conditions, thank your lucky stars. If you did get any of these, you probably wish it didn't happen.

Because bad things due to cannabis haven't happened to you doesn't mean they won't happen to your friend or the vulnerable or unfortunate. Hey, most people don't die in car crashes; but 0.97% do. It doesn't mean it doesn't happen, and it doesn't mean you are not going to drive. It means a wise person is going to *slow down* and be more careful or maybe take the train.

4. *The fourth important concept is:* This is not the marijuana of the 1969 Woodstock generation.
The concentration of THC in marijuana has increased from approximately 2-4% in 1969 to often over 20% today, over 10 times as strong[35, 36]. The pot we smoked in high school in 1969 could just as easily have been floor sweepings, we wouldn't

have known the difference. This increase in potency is associated with higher health risks than in the past[37] and now with edibles, vaping, extracts, and concentrates, the THC can reach over 80%[36]. Plant breeding and cultivation techniques of *Cannabis sativa, Cannabis indica* and specific strains, continues to drive the THC potency higher and higher, while the amount of CBD often declines, depending on the strain. Today's marijuana is not your parents pot, or as the Surgeon General said, "This ain't your mother's marijuana"[38]. If you are a parent and think "I'm a hypocrite if I say little Jimmy can't smoke pot, because I did in high school". He's not smoking what you smoked. Actually, he may not be just smoking weed...he's increasingly more likely vaping, dabbing[39], eating edibles[40, 41], or using concentrates[42], like wax or shatter.

Chapter 4

Marijuana Myths and other important thoughts about Weed

Marijuana is Not Addictive; Marijuana is natural so it can't be bad; Weed is not a gateway drug to harder drugs; There is not enough scientific study of marijuana; Legalization and the public perception of safety; Industry Disinformation; Weed Use Trajectories; Edibles; Poly-Substance Use; Thoughts about Medical Marijuana.

Myths about weed.

Myth 1. Marijuana is Not Addictive

It is clear that in some people, smoking weed can lead to a physical or psychological dependence or addiction, and this shares neurobiological aspects of addiction with other drugs of abuse[43]. From 2002-2017 Cannabis Use Disorder (CUD)[44] "was the most prevalent substance use disorder in North America except alcohol use disorder"[45]. Marijuana dependence and addiction is directly related to the *BIG FOUR*, mentioned above; How early, How often, How much, How strong. Moreover, there is evidence that CUD is more prevalent in males than in females. An excellent discussion of marijuana dependency, addiction, symptoms of withdrawal, and therapies for marijuana addiction can be found in the book, "Marijuana: The unbiased truth about the worlds most popular weed" by Kevin P. Hill M.D[46].

In a study of almost 750,000 people in the United States, among adult cannabis users, the prevalence of a Cannabis Use Disorder diagnosis was 9.3% in 2017[44]. Another report in the *Journal of the American Medical Association-Psychiatry* using the National Survey on Drug Use and Health of over 500,00 respondents in the United States stated that among *past-year* marijuana users ages 12-17, the rate of Cannabis Use Disorder in 2016 was 27.2%[47]. A commonly cited study[48] from 2011 determined the transition to dependence in cannabis users to be 8.9%. By comparison, the same study found a transition to dependence in alcohol users of 22.7%. The variation in the rate of cannabis dependence in different studies is likely due to differences in the people studied, requirements for inclusion in the different studies, and different ways researchers calculate their statistics. Whatever way different research groups calculate it, they find Cannabis Use Disorder.

In a recent review, Ferlund and colleagues[49] describe the biology and physiology of Cannabis Use Disorder and state that CUD "often has its genesis in adolescence and in vulnerable individuals associated with psychiatric co-morbidity, genetic and environmental factors". Cannabis use disorder affects one in six adolescent cannabis users[50]. Symptoms of withdrawal from heavy and prolonged cannabis use have also recently been reviewed[51].

These are the official diagnostic features of Cannabis Use Disorder as described in the Diagnostic and statistical manuals of mental disorders: DSM-5[52]. See anything familiar? Think on these things in relation to your use of weed or those around you.

DSM-5 Diagnostic criteria for Cannabis Use Disorders

A problematic pattern of cannabis use leading to clinically significant impairment or distress as manifested by *at least two* of the following occurring in a 12-month period:

1. Cannabis is often taken in larger amounts over a longer period than was intended.

2. There is a persistent desire or insignificant effort to cut down or control cannabis use.

3. A great deal of time is spent in activities necessary to obtain cannabis, use cannabis, or recover from its effects.

4. Craving or a strong desire to use cannabis.

5. Recurrent cannabis use resulting in a failure to fulfill major obligations at work, school or home.

6. Continued cannabis use despite having persistent or recurrent social or interpersonal problems caused or exacerbated by the effects of cannabis.

7. Important social, occupational or recreational activities are given up or reduced because of cannabis use.

8. Recurrent cannabis use in situations which is physically hazardous.

9. Cannabis use is continued despite knowledge of having persistent or recurrent physical or psychological problems that are unlikely to have been caused or exacerbated by cannabis.

10. Tolerance as defined by either: A) a need for markedly increased amounts of cannabis to achieve intoxication and desired effect, or B) a markedly diminished effect with continued use of the same amount of cannabis.

11. Withdrawal, as manifested by either: A. the characteristic withdrawal symptoms for cannabis, or B. a closer related substance is taken to relieve or avoid withdrawal symptoms.

Myth 2. Marijuana is natural so it can't be bad

Natural is not necessarily safe[53]. Just because something comes from a plant and is considered natural doesn't mean it can't be harmful. The shrub oleander (*Nerium oleander*) can cause cardiac and neuronal symptoms[54]. Wolfsbane (*Aconitum*) contains a fatal neurotoxin[55]. Castor beans contain the deadly toxin ricin. These are a few examples of the many plants that contain alkaloids and other toxic chemicals, which they use for environmental protection or to ward off bacteria, fungus, insects, birds, and mammals. That's why these substances are in the plants. So, just because something is found naturally in plants, that doesn't mean the plant is safe. The same is true of the compounds in marijuana. They are not there to get high. They are most likely in marijuana to ward off predators. In addition, the natural quality of weed can be tainted by unscrupulous growers who may use banned pesticides and other chemicals in the growing and processing of weed that can leave harmful contaminants[56-59]. Natural doesn't always mean safe.

Myth 3. Weed is not a gateway drug to harder drugs.

Not for most people, but it can be...in *some* people. Will it act as a gateway drug in you, maybe not. Might it happen to your friend, maybe[60-62][63, 64]. A seminal scientific study by Denise Kandel published in the journal *Science* in 1975 followed 5,498 students in New York from secondary school through postgraduation. The study defined 4 stages of progression from non-use of drugs to the use of harder drugs. These 4 stages are: beer/wine; to hard liquor/ cigarettes; then marijuana; then other illicit drugs. These are general stages. While some adolescents progress through the stages, many do not[64], with others stopping altogether. A 2020 study[65] of adolescents from alternative high schools in southern California concluded that use of marijuana, tobacco, and alcohol may drive a greater latitude of acceptance toward substance use in general, which may accelerate the transition from gateway drugs to hard drugs.

In a 2015 study of 6,624 people representative of the US population who started cannabis use before using any other drug it was estimated that 44.7% of individuals with lifetime cannabis use progressed to other illicit drug use at some time in their lives[61]. Similarly, in a sample of 10,641 adults, representative of the general population in Australia, the authors noted "In particular, cannabis abuse and dependence were highly associated with increased risks of other substance dependence"[63]. In addition, in a 25 year study following 1,265 New Zealand children, the authors found that "regular or heavy cannabis use was associated with an increased risk of using other illicit drugs, abusing or becoming dependent upon other illicit drugs, and using a wider variety of other illicit drugs"[60].

Animal studies support the human studies, showing that THC can "prime the brain for enhanced responses to other drugs"[2, 66, 67] and this process may affect individuals differently. In a recent study in the journal *Neuropharmacology*, adolescent 6 week old rats of two different genetic backgrounds were given THC or saline for 4 weeks, and then the THC was taken away. Next, the rats were set up to self-administer heroin. One rat strain self administered more heroin if it was first pretreated with THC, whereas the other rat strain self administered less heroin[67], suggesting that different people may be susceptible in different ways to other drugs later in life, depending on their unique genetic backgrounds and their exposure to THC as adolescents.

Myth 4. There is not enough scientific study of marijuana.
There are many common myths about marijuana, and one is that there has not been a lot of scientific study on marijuana and that we can't make important life decisions until "all the facts are

in". That is false. There are currently over 35,000 publications about marijuana in PubMed, the public repository of medical and scientific publications, and that number grows every day. How many have you read? My guess is about *zero*. You are in luck, here is your chance. This book will make it easy. These publications describe the basic science of the effect of THC and other biochemicals found in weed on cells, tissues and organs, as well as more complex outcomes related to brain development, memory, cognition, behavior, psychological conditions such as psychosis, depression and anxiety, as well as societal effects of weed such as effects on education, employment, driving, and violence. Most areas of research in marijuana are growing robustly and there are many research groups committed to expanding the scope and depth of research. Do we need more scientific study of weed? Absolutely, especially well controlled population studies on the effects of weed on adolescents and brain development or studies on the true value of medical marijuana and CBD, beyond the hype. But do we know a lot about weed? Can we make informed personal decisions about our health based on current scientific knowledge? Absolutely.

As legalization and decriminalization efforts around the world go forward, there is an increasing social belief that marijuana is very safe.
It just ain't so, Joe. In a 2019 study[68] from the University of California San Francisco of over 9000 people, scientists studied "statements of misinformation, for example, smoking marijuana has preventative health benefits, secondhand marijuana smoke or use during pregnancy is completely or somewhat safe, and marijuana is not at all addictive". Forty-three percent believed "unsupported claims about marijuana". They found that those people that had gotten information about weed from social media or the internet, the marijuana industry, or friends or relatives were more likely to believe any statement consistent with misinformation about marijuana. Other studies have also

found an increasing belief in the public in the safety of weed in direct contrast to scientific and medical evidence[69-71].

Industry Disinformation

The flow of scientific information between business and industry and the general public is complex and multifaceted. The interpretation and presentation of scientific research can sometimes become bent. By and large, business and industry spokespeople are on the up and up, they speak the truth, or at least what they think is the truth. It is their job to enthusiastically promote their industry. However, as the Union of Concerned Scientists describes, there are times when "business interests deceive, misinform, and buy influence at the expense of public health and safety"[72]. Industry spokespeople can sometimes minimize the health risk to their industry's advantage at the expense of public health. Whether it is cigarettes and cancer in the 1950s and 60s, environmental toxins in the 70s and 80s, climate change in the 90s and 2000s, or unhealthy food...all the time; there is constant pressure from monied interests to promote their interests, and influence legislation for those who are paying the bills. The Cannabis industry is no different. With billions of dollars up for grabs, health risks are minimized by industry advocates and the science of health and cannabis can and will get distorted[73]. It would be wise not to get health advice from Cannabis industry spokespeople or websites funded by the Cannabis industry.

Weed Use Trajectories

Scientists like to put things into categories. One useful way to look at the way people use marijuana is to put weed usage patterns into age trajectories[74-77]. How do different people use weed at different times over their life. None at all? Do they just use a little every now and then? Do they use a lot when they are young but it trails off, using less and less, eventually stopping? Do they use a lot regularly and keep at it?

As shown in figure 2, in 2019 a Canadian research group reported a study[78] of 662 youth from age 15 to 28 in the Victoria Healthy Youth Survey. They identified 5 classes of weed users; abstainers, occasional users, decreasers, increasers, and chronic users.

Figure 2. Latent classes of marijuana use from 15 to 28 years of age

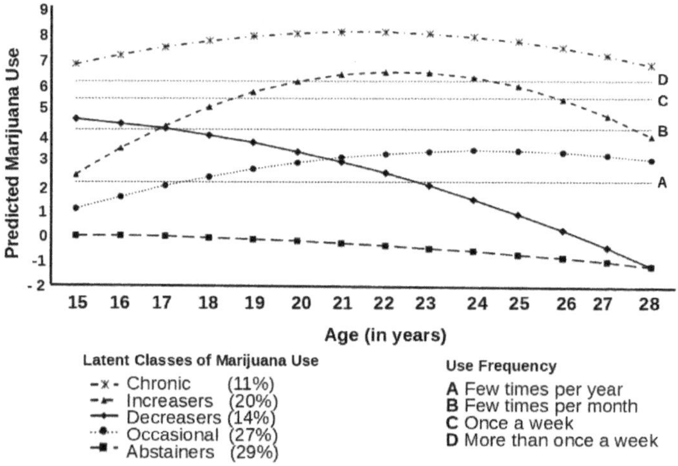

Latent Classes of Marijuana Use
-x- Chronic   (11%)
-ᴧ- Increasers   (20%)
-◆- Decreasers   (14%)
...◆... Occasional (27%)
-■- Abstainers   (29%)

Use Frequency
A Few times per year
B Few times per month
C Once a week
D More than once a week

Similarly, a research group at the University of Chicago studied[79] over 1,200 9th and 10th graders and followed them over the next six years. They identified four trajectories of marijuana use from age 14 to 23, Low, Medium, High, and Escalating. In the first three trajectories, marijuana use tapered off in the early twenties.

In 2016 researchers from Wake Forest School of Medicine reported a study of 2,500 college students[80] from eleven different colleges, and their cannabis use measured at six time points over their college experience. They identified five trajectories of cannabis use; non-users, infrequent users, decreasing users, increasing users, and frequent users. One finding was, "all four marijuana use groups reported significantly lower GPAs, on average, than non-users. Even students who used marijuana infrequently exhibited lower academic performance." They concluded that, "Decreasing and frequent marijuana users were both less likely to be currently enrolled in college as of senior year and were less likely to plan to graduate on time, suggesting that students who frequently use marijuana early in their college career are most at risk of not completing college and delaying graduation." This strengthened previous similar findings on the academic consequences of marijuana use[81].

Another group of scientists studied almost 6,000 young Swiss men[82] with Cannabis Use Disorder at age 20, then accessed them again at 21.5 and 25 years old. They were classified into four groups based on their usage of weed; stable-low (88.2%, decreasing (5.2%, stable-high (2.6% and increasing (4.0%.

As compared to the stable-low trajectory, the stable-high and decreasing trajectories were associated with increased major depression severity, attention deficit hyperactivity disorder severity, antisocial personality disorder severity, poor relationship with parents, number of friends with drug problems, neuroticism-anxiety, and less sociability.

Does your weed use fit into a trajectory? Do you stop using weed after the novelty has worn off? Think about it. Similar weed trajectories, described below, have been described for other life outcomes such as education and employment.

Edibles

Edibles are food products infused with marijuana or purified THC. Important things to remember about marijuana edibles are that they take a longer time to kick in than smoking weed, and the concentration and dosing may not be easy to figure out. With a joint you sort of know how much you are getting and how quickly it will take effect, not so much with an edible. Don't eat an edible, then 30 minutes later say "hey...it's not working... then eat more. That is a recipe for disaster.[83]. Jonathan Zipursky and colleagues at the University of Toronto suggest these 5 Things To Know About Edible Cannabis[84]

1. More than 40% of North American nonmedical cannabis users consume edibles.

2. Edibles have a long latency period and duration of action. (Which means they take longer to affect you and may last longer)

3. Unfamiliarity with edible dosing and difficulties in dividing edibles can result in unintentional overdose.

4. Psychiatric and cardiovascular complications are more likely with edibles.

5. Unintentional exposure to edibles is particularly dangerous for children.

Poly-Substance Use
Teens go to a party, or hang with their friends, maybe drink alcohol *AND* smoke weed, or do other drugs. Or maybe they are becoming addicted to vaping nicotine *AND* vape THC or smoke weed *AND* binge drink alcohol. You know this happens, I know this happens, everybody knows this happens. Bottom line is...bad plus bad equals really bad.

In a recent study of almost 75,000 high school students in Canada, "of those who used substances, approximately half (53%) reported using two or more substances. E-cigarette vaping was most prevalent (28%), followed by current binge drinking (17%) and cannabis use (13%)"[85].

In the scientific literature this is called Poly-Substance Use. There are multiple research studies reporting a link between mental health issues and other problems associated with poly-substance use. Many published reports have found that psychiatric symptoms, including depression and anxiety[86-91] are associated with increased risk of poly-substance use[85].

An increasingly popular way to use both nicotine and cannabis is vaping through e-cigarettes, especially for adolescents and young adults. The lung injuries that have been associated with contaminants in vaping systems have been well documented[92]. As noted by the U.S. Centers for Disease Control and Prevention as of February 18, 2020, there have been a total of 2,807 hospitalizations including 68 deaths associated with E-cigarette, or Vaping, product use-Associated Lung Injury (EVALI) [93]. Vaping is a particularly potent way to get both nicotine and THC into your system. One in ten students reported ever vaping cannabis in a study of 2,835 high schoolers mostly between the ages of 14–18 years in North Carolina[94], a significant number of those students vaped nicotine as well.

Other reports of harm related to cannabis and poly-substance use include Cognitive function impairment[95] with weed and alcohol, alterations of brain white matter integrity[96] with cannabis and binge drinking, A special "Shout Down" (opposite of shout out) goes out for mixing weed, alcohol, or other drugs and driving[97]. In a recent study, traffic collisions tripled when drivers drove under the influence of both cannabis and alcohol as compared to either one alone[98].

Thoughts about Medical Marijuana, Cannabinoids, and Pharmaceutical preparations of Cannabinoids.
Although this book is not specifically about medical marijuana, here are some thoughts on that topic to help put that issue into perspective. There is mixed scientific evidence about the efficacy of medical marijuana[99]. This includes early preliminary

evidence for beneficial effects in sleep[100,101] anxiety[102], appetite, neuropathic pain[101,103], pain associated with cancer, spasticity in multiple sclerosis[104], obsessive compulsive disorder[105], Tourette syndrome[106], liver disorders[107-109], headache[110], and nausea[111-114], among other conditions. In almost all cases, possible benefits occur at low doses or short term use while the potential for harm creeps up with high doses or chronic use.

In many cases there are studies and systematic reviews that report negative results or harm for cannabis use in these same conditions; including depression and anxiety[115], sleep, and pain[116], to name a few. In 2019 a systematic review of 1,972 scientific papers[117] on medical marijuana, emphasizing pain management, the authors concluded., "Many reviews were unable to provide firm conclusions on the effectiveness of medical cannabis, and results of reviews were mixed. Mild adverse effects were frequently but inconsistently reported, and it is possible that harms may outweigh benefits. Evidence from longer-term, adequately powered, and methodologically sound Randomized Controlled Trials exploring different types of cannabis-based medicines is required for conclusive recommendations.

Most carefully controlled experimental scientific studies of cannabis for medical purposes do not use recreational marijuana in any form, such as smoked or edibles. The composition and concentration of cannabinoids in recreational marijuana varies widely. They simply add too much variability and noise in the data. Instead, the studies use standardized pharmaceutical grade synthetic or purified THC or CBD, or other cannabinoids, such as Dronabinol[118]; a chemically synthesized THC, Savitex[119]; a 1:1 mixture of THC:CBD, Nabilone[120]; a THC analog, or Epidiolex[121]; a purified preparation of CBD. Large population studies that aggregate data from many thousands of people may collect data from users who use different types of medical marijuana products or recreational marijuana, but this could introduce wide variation which tends to mess with the statistics. Going into a cannabis shop and buying some OG Kush bud for anxiety bears little resemblance to the THC or other cannabinoids used in carefully controlled studies.

Having said all that, there are many compelling anecdotal stories of individuals obtaining benefit from medical applications of cannabis or cannabis products. Which gets back to how people are different. There is much more careful scientific work to be done.

Chapter 5
Biological, Biochemical, and Genetic Basics

Tetrahydrocannabinol, THC and Cannabidiol, CBD; Tolerance to THC; Common Genetics and Weed; DNA: The Long Stringy Stuff; Four Important Genes; Epigenetics; Cytochrome P450s: Cannabis, Prescription Drug interactions and Metabolism.

Tetrahydrocannabinol and Cannabidiol

The main psychoactive chemical in marijuana is delta-9-tetrahydrocannabinol, also known as **THC**[122]. It is a cannabinoid, a chemical found in cannabis. THC exists in the Cannabis plant for protection against attack from bacteria, fungi, viruses, and other creatures. THC is one of at least 113 other cannabinoids found in Cannabis[123]. When you smoke, eat, or vape weed, the THC is broken down, mainly in your liver, into over 100 metabolites, some of which are psychoactive or have other biological activities. It is then excreted in your feces and urine[122]. THC is not naturally found in your body. THC is responsible for the high from weed. It promotes dependence, impairs cognition, and is associated with hallucinations, paranoid ideas and psychotic disorders[124].

Figure 3. Molecular Structure of THC and CBD

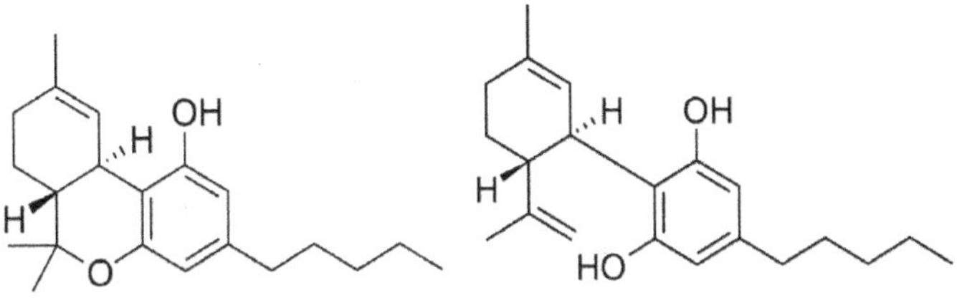

THC   CBD

Cannabidiol or **CBD**[125] is the other major cannabinoid found in marijuana. It is remarkably similar in structure to THC[122]. CBD is non-psychoactive, does not produce a "high", and is being investigated for different therapeutic applications[126]. It does not adversely effect cognition, and does not promote dependence. CBD is not associated with psychosis and may, in fact, have anti-psychotic properties[124]. The relative proportions of THC to CBD are different in different strains of weed and this ratio is important in medical applications[127]. The relative proportions of THC versus CBD in a Cannabis plant are in balance since they are made from the same molecular precursor, Cannabigerol[128]. So the more THC a plant makes, the less CBD, or the more CBD, the less THC. Of course, in a prepared product like an edible or an extract, that ratio can be artificially altered.

Generally, the many years of plant breeding of different strains of *Cannabis sativa*[129] have maximized the concentration of THC over CBD, while strains of *Cannabis indica*[130] and hybrids between *sativa* and *indica* tend to have a more balanced ratio of CBD to THC. For example, the *C. sativa* strain Shangrila contains 22% THC and 0.05% CBD, while the hybrid Candida (CD-1) has 20% CBD and 1% THC.

An important biochemical quality of THC as opposed to say alcohol is that THC is lipophilic; oily and soluble in fat...your fat, as opposed to alcohol which is soluble in water. You pee out alcohol within about 24 hours, while you retain THC in your body, largely in your fat, from 4 to 6 days[131]. THC can be found in a urine drug test up to a month after use. So if you smoke weed regularly, you always have some THC in your system. Do you know what organ is 60% fat? *Your brain.*

THC binds to receptors on the surface of cells in your brain and immune system called Cannabinoid Receptors[132], CB1 (the gene is known as CNR1[133]) and CB2 (the gene is known as CNR2[134,135]). These receptors are a part of the endocannabinoid system, a natural biochemical pathway involved in many cell functions, very importantly in reward, motivation, sleep[136], and pleasure pathways centered on the neurotransmitter dopamine[137, 138]. Two natural compounds your body makes in the endocannabinoid system include anandamide[139] and 2-arachidonoylglycerol. These bind to cannabinoid receptors and signal biochemical pathways, including dopamine pathways in cells. THC hijacks the endocannabinoid system by binding to these receptors and competes with the anandamide found in your brain. In the short run, THC overstimulates the receptors and the endocannabinoid system, but when you use weed chronically, THC down-regulates CB1 receptors and blunts the dopamine response system[140-143].

This is key. Down-regulating the receptors and blunting the system means that using weed a lot makes the dopamine response system in your brain less responsive. This is part of the reason why chronic users get less of a high over time. This can lead some people to smoke more weed each time or cause them to switch to more potent cannabis strains to maintain a certain level of buzz[144].

Dopamine is a very important hormone neurotransmitter[137]. Dopamine pathways are central to the many different effects of weed. For example, dopamine is involved in signaling cells to express complex gene programs. When neurons are triggered, say through the CB1 receptor, they release neurotransmitters, stimulating other neurons to produce dopamine, which travels to the next neuron, thus stimulating that cell. This creates a cascade of activation along neuronal pathways. Both the dopamine system in your brain and how THC hijacks and manipulates your dopamine pathways are complex. Dopaminergic pathways are involved in many important higher order brain functions, such as executive functions[145], appetite, learning, reward, emotion, pleasure, motivation, and neuroendocrine control[146]. Although study of these complex biological processes is ongoing, scientific evidence of the effects of weed on neuronal signaling continues to become clearer.

Brain imaging and other studies show that chronic use of weed may alter multiple biochemical pathways, including dopamine signaling pathways, neuronal circuitry, and metabolism in the frontal cortex, dorsal striatum, nucleus accumbens, substantia nigra, ventral tegmental area,[147, 148], and other regions of the brain[149]. These regions of the brain are important in the mesocorticolimbic pathway[150, 151], a major dopamine pathway in the brain, also known as the reward pathway, influencing motivation, desire, and pleasure. These effects of cannabis on the brain occur in humans and is strongly supported by highly specific controlled studies in rats.

Alteration of dopamine pathways is a key feature of many of the long term negative effects of Cannabis. Weed may make you feel good for today and may lower today's anxiety, but there is evidence that over time, chronic activation of dopamine signaling pathways slowly blunts your dopamine release path-ways, contributing to an increase in negative emotionality[140], dependence, addiction, increases in apathy[152], and increases in anxiety and depression.

Tolerance to THC

Tolerance to THC is what happens when you have a need for markedly increased amounts of cannabis to achieve the same high or a diminished effect with continued use of the same amount of cannabis. It is a neurobiological process that can occur with chronic use. It can be thought of as "building up a resistance to weed", where you need more and more to get the same buzz. It occurs in humans and in test animals[143, 153, 154]. Foundational scientific studies of marijuana tolerance in humans suggest that prolonged use of weed can reduce subjective and physiologic responses[155] to cannabis intoxication. Tolerance to THC can be a milepost on the way to dependence.

Common Genetics and Weed

Many people in the general public think about the genetic risk with marijuana *wrong* and they run a big risk in getting it wrong. It is a common misconception that the unfortunate few have the bad gene, thinking "I don't have that gene, that's not me, bummer for you!". The media contributes to this misinformation since they very often use the wrong terminology, almost always reporting," This person has *the gene* for this or that." The fact is, most people have the *same* genes, pretty much, give or take. What's important is we have different *variants* of the same genes, that is where the action is, gene variants.

Here is the deal. For the purposes of this discussion, there are two types of human genetics. **Rare single gene disorders** with gene mutations having strong disease causing effects. (Think Huntington's disease, Sickle cell anemia, Tay sachs disease, Dwarfism etc.) They are very rare, they can occur roughly from 1 in 1000, to less than 1 in 100,000 people. That means it is very unlikely that anyone with these rare gene mutations works where you work or goes to your school or lives on your street. These mutations are fairly new in the human population, like up to hundreds of years old. This is the genetics of Gregor Mendel[156] or Mendelian genetics. As far as many health conditions are concerned, this is most likely *not* you. This is definitely *not* the genetics of substance abuse. The other type of human genetics, the *important* one in the case of weed, is the genetics of **common complex quantitative traits**[157]. This involves multiple genes with many variations with small disease effects, and interactions with environmental factors, such as weed.

DNA: The Long Stringy Stuff

Your DNA contains strings of nucleotides (A,T,C or G) which code for GENES. When needed, your GENES make different RNAs, RNA codes for PROTEINS which are made up of amino acids. PROTEINS are building blocks for things like enzymes, and structural proteins. PROTEINS do stuff, like control biochemical pathways or help build cells, organs and tissues.

Genes have two names, the long formal name and the short gene symbol. It's kind of like company names and their stock symbols, like Microsoft, (MSFT) or Apple, (AAPL). There are at least 12 important Genes that we know about, that have multiple common variants in the population that have been associated with cannabis disorders. There are certainly many more we don't know about. These may make you respond differently to weed than the next guy or girl. It is most likely that you may have some of these gene variants.

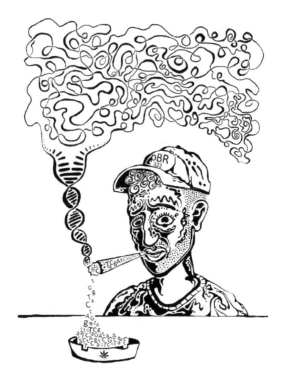

These genetic variations in your DNA, involve single nucleotide polymorphisms (SNPs) These are single letter differences (A,T,C, or G) in the nucleotides in your DNA, shared within different ethnic groups. These are the type of variations that are tested for by the new direct to consumer genetic testing companies, such as 23andMe, or Ancestry.com, where you spit in a tube and mail it off. These variants are usually fairly common. Look to the left and look to the right, then look at yourself. Everyone you look at is carrying some of these gene variants.

Each SNP is given a reference number or "rs number", which stands for "Reference SNP cluster ID. They look like this: rs12345(X), where X is either A, T, C, or G. You can have an A, T, C, or G in the DNA at each one of these positions. There are millions of these SNP variants all over the more than 3 billion nucleotides in your personal human genome; and so it is with everybody. But yet, we are still 99.9% identical in our DNA to the next random person and 99% identical to chimpanzees. Mind blowing, ain't it! It's one thing that makes you...you. Many of these SNPs do not result in a protein change. They can affect regulation of the genome in other ways, or just be hanging out silently. These variants are found in SNP genetic databases, such as SNPedia[153].

What's in *YOUR* DNA?

For the nerdy out there, I have included a link below to a list of all the 29 gene variants with some evidence of an association to Cannabis use, and a description on ways to research your genetic variants. https://whoadude-the-book.com/how-to-search-your-snps/

If you have taken a commercial DNA test, like Ancestry.com, or 23andMe, it is possible to find out your nucleotides (A,T,C, or G) at the risk variants or SNPs for these genes.

Unlike rare single gene mutations, these SNP gene variants are usually very ancient in the human population, like millions of years. We often share them with our closest primate ancestors[159]. Our own personal collection of these variants make each one of us a little bit different than the next person. Most common chronic medical conditions that are frequent in families involve multiple genetic variants of small effect related to complex traits. These conditions often have a range of severity, instead of yes/no. Things like Type 2 diabetes, obesity, auto-immune disorders, many mental health conditions, and yes substance abuse. This health risk is not strongly genetically determined as it is in rare single gene disorders. The health risks related to common variants is greatly influenced by the environment through what are called gene-environment inter-actions. In this case environment doesn't mean the outdoors...

like trees and clouds and climate. It means what you eat, smoke, consume, get exposed to, and do.

It's important to know that having these gene variants doesn't mean you are going to get the disorder, it means you might be predisposed to the disorder under certain circumstances. It means you...*could* get it if things don't go your way, or if you don't take care of yourself. These types of conditions all involve small genetic variants that interact over time with environmental factors, such as diet, exercise, infections, and things you ingest; like weed. You have a say in the process, you can't control your genetics, but you can control the environmental triggers, such as substances you consume. All people carry some of the variants of genes that little-by-little contribute and add up to complex health risk, since they are important in many different medical contexts. This means you.

The gene variants important in health risks in marijuana *are not in your genome because of marijuana*. These human gene variants have generally been positively selected through evolution and are related to things like personality, pleasure, mental health, impulsivity, pain response, memory, cognition, and normal complex brain functions. The functions of most of the variants are still unknown. Marijuana hijacks the gene variants that you have and may contribute to your individual weed related health risk. Weed is a gene variant hijacker.

Impulsivity and Gene Variants: Is it a Deer or is it a Saber Toothed Tiger?

The ancient gene variants, or SNPs, that marijuana influences are *not* in your genome because of marijuana. They are there for some other ancient, often out of context reason. It's true for many common gene SNPs. Take impulsivity for instance[160] The CNR1 gene variants, rs2023239, rs1049353, rs806368, which marijuana hijacks, may have an influence on being impulsive[161]. Say you are a cave man or cave woman 50,000 years ago[162]. You are snoozing in the cave with your clan. You hear a rustling outside. You impulsively jump up to investigate. Your more cautious, less impulsive friend Grog keeps snoozing. Is it a deer or a Saber toothed tiger? If it is a deer, you could feed your clan for a week (and your genes might get passed on, *Woo Hoo!*). If it is a Saber toothed tiger, it might eat you. (Bummer dude, it was a Saber toothed tiger). Flash forward 50,000 years. In a modern context, you and your less spontaneous more cautious friend George are at a party. Someone says, "try a hit of this killer Bro Grimms Cinderella 99 bud". You say, thank you mama!. Your friend says, no thanks...I'm cool; Impulsivity? Could be due to something random, could be related to gene variants, out of evolutionary context. Impulsivity gene variants play out in many aspects of life.

If you or a relative, like a brother, sister, parent, cousin, aunt or uncle has a problem with substance abuse, including alcoholism, or mental health issues such as bipolar disorder, depression, anxiety, or schizophrenia, there is a very good chance some of these common small-effect risk gene variants found in complex traits related to brain function are carried in you, your family, or your kids, and are just hanging out doing their normal job.

A 2020 study in the journal *Psychological Medicine* reported that 152 gene variants[163] were simultaneously shared by both substance use, including cannabis, *and* psychiatric disorders including; ADHD, anorexia, bipolar disorder, major depressive disorder and schizophrenia. And again, these variants, which typically cause tiny effects and usually have unknown function, don't give you a disease or condition. They may predispose you to a condition. They also may impart positive attributes. That is usually why they have evolved, or they may increase your risk for different health conditions in today's world, accelerated by environmental factors...like weed. Your friend or the guy down the street, may not have these gene variants and they might be able to smoke a big spliff every day, no problem, but you...not so much.

Four Genes important in susceptibility to Cannabis

Cannabinoid receptor 1—CNR1

The Cannabinoid receptor 1[133, 164] is a protein receptor in the endocannabinoid system found on the surface of cells in the brain and central nervous system, as well as other cells and tissues of the body. The gene that encodes this receptor goes by the initials CNR1, whereas the protein product goes by CB1. THC binds to CB1 and signals the dopamine pathway and other important biochemical pathways. The gene CNR1 has over 16 different genetic variants in the population. The effects of most of these different forms are unknown, and many will be benign, normal variants with no or little effect. However there are some variants of CNR1 that can make you susceptible to cannabis dependence while the alternate type at that position may protect you against harmful effects. Hopfer and colleagues[165] reported that the common variant rs806368[166] "was significantly associated with cannabis problem use" in the people they tested. There is evidence that at least three of the variants in CNR1 (rs806368(C), rs1049353(A)and rs1049353(G)) work together in complex ways to influence your health of a number of conditions like susceptibility to cannabis[167-169], alcohol[170], nicotine[171], cocaine addiction[172, 173], obesity[174], anger-hostility,[175] impulsivity[161], and even PTSD[176]. Some studies have not found any associations with cannabis use[177]. More work is needed to nail down what is going on.

The risk variants for cannabis use and CNR1 SNP rs806368 is C/C, and for rs1049353 is C/C. This a weak association at best and may vary in different ethnic groups. I am personally type T/T at the SNP rs806368, and C/C at rs1049353; which is weakly associated with cannabis susceptibility risk.

Catechol-O-methyltransferase—COMT

The neurotransmitter dopamine is broken down by the enzyme catechol-O-methyltransferase or COMT[178]. The neurotransmitter dopamine is involved in many important aspects of neuronal and brain functions including pleasure and reward motivated behavior[137]. Everybody has the COMT gene, its just that different people have different versions or variants of the COMT gene. Some versions are found more often in people with risk for different conditions such as depression, bipolar disorder, ADHD as well as cannabis use neuropsychological impairment[13, 179]. One of the many variants of COMT, with official designation rs4680, can code for either the amino acid Valine (VAL) or Methionine (MET) at amino acid position 158 in the COMT protein. This is coded for by either a G or an A nucleotide in your DNA. Since you carry two copies of each gene, one from mom and one from dad, you can be one of three posibilities at this position; G/G nucleotides coding for VAL/VAL amino acids; or G/A and VAL/MET or A/A coding for MET/MET. MET carriers have less of the enzyme COMT and therefore dopamine is broken down more slowly in their prefrontal cortex in the brain, than VAL carriers, resulting in higher levels of dopamine. This VAL/MET variant of COMT is the basis for the well known Warrior/Worrier phenotype[180]. Interestingly, the VAL COMT variant has been shown to be increased in mixed-martial arts fighters[180]. The risk variant for cannabis and COMT SNP rs4680 is G/G. This G/G risk form is found in about 30-50% of the general population depending on ethnic origin[186]. I personally am A/A, coding for the amino acids Met/Met for COMT variant rs4680, the worrier phenotype (big surprise), higher dopamine levels, not associated with bad outcomes in cannabis use.

In a study in 2005, researchers at King's College London noted that, "Cannabis use in adolescents was associated with increased risk of schizophrenia related disorders in adulthood among

COMT Val158Val individuals and, to a lesser extent, among Met/Val individuals but not among Met/Met individuals"[181].

Depending on what ethnic group you are related to, about 30-50% of people carry the risk form, VAL/VAL and 30 to 50% carry the medium risk form VAL/MET. Only ~8-24% of people carry the low risk form. So, when you think pot and genetics, don't think "that's not me", instead think "that could be me". Bad outcomes have been associated with COMT at the rs4680 position and cannabis use in multiple studies[31, 182-186].

Dopamine receptor D2—DRD2

Dopamine receptors[187, 188, 189, 190] are a family of proteins found on the surface of neurons and other tissues that are involved in the complex signaling of dopamine[137], the neurotransmitter that is central to cognition, memory, reward and pleasure pathways and other biological processes. Gene variants in dopamine receptors have been associated with ADHD, pathological gambling, schizophrenia, as well as drug and alcohol abuse, among other things. Strangely, dopamine receptors have been shown to be important in vomiting[191] (see Chapter 9). Dopamine receptors are also the target of antipsychotic medications such as risperidone and haldoperidol.

There is emerging and conflicting evidence that gene variants of DRD2 are associated with cannabis abuse[192]. The main effect of DRD2 genetic variants may be on a general susceptibility to psychosis, while cannabis kicks that susceptibility into high gear. A study from King's College London in 2015 of 758 individuals showed that a variant, rs1076560, of the DRD2 genotype may modulate the psychosis inducing effect of cannabis use[193]. For this variant of DRD2, the high-risk form is T and the low-risk form is G. (So you can be T/T, T/G, or G/G). Healthy individuals carrying the T form of this DRD2 variant did have an increase in schizophrenic like behavior, called schizotypy, as compared to both cannabis users and non-users who had the G/G. But daily cannabis users, with the T variant had a 5-fold increase in the odds of psychosis compared to G/G carriers. This DRD2 variant is also associated with an increased risk of alcoholism[194].

I am personally a G/G for DRD2 variant rs1076560, the low-risk variant. The T/T version of this variant for DRD2 is not very frequent (<2 %) in people of European descent, but is higher in Asians and people of Mexican ancestry[195].

Another important gene variant for Dopamine Receptor 2 or DRD2, is rs6277, also referred to as C957T, which results in an amino acid change in the protein. Although it is controversial[196], there is evidence that this variant may be involved in brain executive function and working memory[197, 198], as well as associated with neuroticism, risk taking, and schizophrenia[199]. A study in 2012[200] found evidence that this variant, DRD2 rs6277 interacted with variants in the PENK gene to influence neuroticism which in turn resulted in a 9-fold increase risk for cannabis dependence.

CC is the risk genotype for DRD2 rs6277 for schizophrenia, and possibly for neuroticism. It is found at a frequency of 17.5% in people with Northern and Western European descent as studied in Utah, and in considerably higher frequency in Asians[201].

Fatty-Acid Amide Hydrolase
Fatty-acid amide hydrolase (FAAH)[202] is a protein enzyme in cell membranes that breaks down molecules such as the two signaling molecules that normally bind to the CB1 cannabinoid receptor, anandamide and 2-AG. FAAH is involved in the regulation of pain[203] and stress[213]. Laboratory mice that lack the FAAH gene show a reduced sensitivity to pain[202].

A recent report[204] described a woman with a DNA mutation in the FAAH gene that resulted in a reduced amount of FAAH protein, making her insensitive to pain, such as pain due to frequent cuts and burns. This was due to an inability to degrade anandamide.

FAAH has been studied in relation to cannabis and substance abuse and the endocannabinoid pathways found in the brain and other tissues. A study from 2002 showed that for the FAAH variant rs324420, a 4.9 times higher risk of combined street drug use and problem drug/alcohol use in carriers of the A/A type than non-carriers. They also demonstrated that this variant, when examined experimentally, produced an FAAH enzyme with significantly increased sensitivity to protein degradation[205].

Additional studies have shown other aspects[206] of FAAH in the context of cannabis[207]; including Cannabis Use Disorder[208,209], craving[209,210] and withdrawal[209,211] as well as new approaches for treatment[208]. The studies on FAAH are complex and more work needs to be done to further define the role of this enzyme and its genetic variants and the relationship to cannabis use.

The high-risk variant for FAAH rs324420 is A/A. The rs324420 A/A risk variant is found in about 4-15% of the population depending on ethnic origin[214]. I personally am type C/C at the FAAH variant rs324420, which does not confer risk for drug use.

Genetics is complicated. Some investigators do not find similar associations with cannabis and these gene variants[215] or the same researchers don't consistently find associations among different population groups for the same gene variants[216]. We only know a little about a small number of genes. We don't know very much at all about the rest of the over ~23,000 genes in your genome. There are almost certainly genes that affect your response to drugs and your psychological well-being that we know nothing about.

There are other aspects of your genome biology related to genes that can be affected by cannabis such as epigenetics, chromatin, and metabolism.

Epigenetics: why it's both interesting and important.

Epi- is from the Greek for "upon or above". Epigenetic processes[217, 218, 219] can modify the letters of your DNA; your A,T,C, and Gs, without actually changing out the letters. Scientists are learning more and more about how DNA can be altered without directly changing the letters of your genetic code. These modifications can affect gene regulation, non-coding RNA levels, or change chromatin[220]; how the DNA is packed into tight coils. One important example of epigenetics is called DNA methylation, where a methyl group (one carbon and three hydrogens) is added to the nucleotide C by enzymes, to make methyl-C. These patterns can change at many places in your genome, and they can occur due to many different factors; such as exercise, aging, and disease but also with drugs. including cannabis. These patterns can change how your genes are turned on and turned off, how much RNA is made from a gene, and subsequently how much protein is made. These patterns may change back to their original state, but the amazing thing is that they can be inherited without changing the basic sequence of your A, T, G, or Cs! What that means, is that you can alter your DNA (or the DNA of a fetus if you are pregnant), which can affect your gene function, *and* it can be passed on to your kids, all without having what is thought to be a classical genetic predisposition. The effects of epigenetic changes in the offspring of mothers that used cannabis and other drugs in utero was recently reviewed for both humans and in supporting animal studies[221,222] It is very early days in the study of epigenetics in general and epigenetics and cannabis use. Much scientific study needs to be done, but the implications of epigenetics are vast.

Cytochrome P450s: Cannabis, Prescription Drug Interactions and Metabolism.

Your liver is the organ that metabolizes and breaks down toxins or natural compounds to be reused or excreted. A major way this happens is through a superfamily of protein enzymes in the liver coded for by 57 genes called the cytochrome P450s[223]. They go by the symbols, CYP1A1, CYP1A2, etc. Different variants of these genes determine whether someone is a fast or slow metabolizer of various prescription drugs. The rate of drug metabolism in the liver alters the effective level of those drugs in the blood. Most people don't know the status of their individual CYP gene variants and whether they are fast or slow metabolizers of a particular drug. Your CYP profile can impact the way that THC is metabolized in the liver[224, 225, 226]. What that means is that if you take a hit of weed, it might stay in your system a lot longer than in your friends system.

Importantly, cannabinoids can also change the levels or activities of cytochrome P450 enzymes and thus can affect the way and the rate that these enzymes break down prescription drugs you may take. You may think you are taking a certain amount of a prescription drug, but due to the affect of cannabinoids and your CYP gene variant status, the concentration of that drug in your blood may vary widely. This may alter the way that the drug treats the condition for which you were taking the prescription drug in the first place.

THC increases the levels of the enzyme CYP1A2. This can theoretically decrease blood concentrations of a number of common prescription drugs, such as clozapine, duloxetine, naproxen, cyclobenzaprine, olanzapine, haloperidol, and chlorpromazine[224, 225, 226].

CBD is a potent inhibitor of the liver enzymes CYP3A4 and CYP2D6. CYP3A4 metabolizes about a quarter of all drugs. CBD may increase blood concentrations of macrolides, calcium channel blockers, benzodiazepines, cyclosporine, sildenafil (Viagra), antihistamines, haloperidol, antiretrovirals, and some statins. CYP2D6 metabolizes many antidepressants, so CBD may increase blood concentrations of SSRIs, tricyclic antidepressants, antipsychotics, beta blockers and opioids[226]. Also, the use of cannabinoids may alter the level of warfarin[227], affecting blood clotting; theophylline, affecting asthma; clobazam, affecting seizures; and valproate affecting seizures and bipolar disorder, among other drugs[228].

Chapter 6

Brain Stuff

Brain Development and Marijuana; Brain Imaging, Cognition, Memory, and IQ.

The human brain is generally thought to be the most complex organ in the human body[229]. Dolphins[230] and elephants also have complex brains and, in fact, have bigger brains than we do, so don't go around being all superior and such. The brain consists of the cerebrum (the big gray part with all the folds), the brainstem (the knob that attaches to the spinal cord) and the cerebellum (the gob stuck on the back). These three parts and the spinal cord make up the central nervous system. Each main part of the brain has many subregions and structures, which have specialized functions and specific jobs. Then you have all the nerves and related things that run to and from the brain and spinal cord to all your organs and muscles. That's your peripheral nervous system.

From the instant a human egg is fertilized, development begins in utero and unfolds a complex program of genes being turned on, cells dividing, complex tissues and organs being built, and connections being established between systems within the body. That process rolls on unabated after birth and continues through childhood and adolescence into young adulthood[231]. A major and essential part of that process is brain development[232, 233, 234]. Brain development is a stepwise process that builds individual parts, such as the hippocampus, prefrontal cortex, and the medula oblongata, with over 86 billion neurons, and creating neuronal connections through dendritic and axon growth, synaptogenesis[235, 236], arborization[237] and many other complex processes. The creation of connections between neurons in the brain is driven by experience and learning. The process continues through adolescence into young adulthood until around age 24. An important late-stage phenomena, which occurs well into our early 20s, is synaptic pruning, in which unneeded neuronal connections are trimmed away, resulting in the mature brain[238].

REMEMBER THIS: *Brain development is a programmed stepwise process that doesn't stop. If you screw it up, there is no going back. There are no do-overs.*

Brain Imaging

The study of brain development considers how the brain grows in volume and complexity, and looks at it functionally. One way to study brain structure and function is with imaging technologies such as magnetic resonance imaging (MRI)[239], computed tomography scanning (CT)[240], and fMRI (functional magnetic resonance imaging)[241]. These imaging tools produce and measure 2D or 3D images of size or volume of regions of the brain that you can then compare under different conditions. fMRI produces images based on relative activity of brain regions based on blood flow or energy usage. Quite often these images highlight regions to count pixels on images. These numbers are converted to colors on the computer, which correspond to regions of high or low brain activity.

There has been conflicting data on whether weed changes the volume or function of brain structures. However, as technology and analytical methods have improved, imaging-based evidence of alterations in the brain is accumulating[242, 243]. Early CT scanning of chronic cannabis users did not show evidence of structural alterations in the brain. However, early CT machines had a limited ability to get data from soft tissue. Using more recent imaging approaches, multiple independent groups have documented atrophy in the hippocampus and parahippocampus associated with chronic cannabis use[244-249]. A brain imaging study[250] in 2015 from Harvard, the University of Cincinnati and the University of Wisconsin tested 59 young adults between the ages of 18 and 25, and demonstrated that marijuana users had significantly smaller medial orbitofrontal cortex (mOFC) volumes (that's in the prefrontal cortex) and inferior parietal volumes. The inferior parietal lobule[251] of the brain is involved in the perception of emotions in facial stimuli, interpretation of sensory information, language, mathematical operations, and body image. These authors[250] concluded that "smaller mOFC volumes among marijuana users suggest disruption of typical neurodevelopmental processes associated with regular marijuana use for both (males and females)".

In other studies, a meta-analysis of multiple neuroimaging studies in healthy volunteers from King's College London consistently showed a smaller hippocampus in cannabis users as compared to nonusers[252], while an MRI study from Australia showed no effect on cortical regions due to cannabis use[253]. A preliminary positron emission tomography (PET) study from 2020 compared people diagnosed with cannabis use disorder versus healthy controls, and showed lower synaptic density in people with cannabis use disorder[254].

Cognition, Memory, and IQ

Does THC mess up your ability to think, reason, and remember things? How are these cognitive process affected while you are high? And how are they affected in the long run, with chronic heavy marijuana use? Recall that in Chapter 4 I introduced cannabinoid receptors, which bind THC. These receptors are widely distributed in the brain, including in areas that influence cognition, thinking, motivation, attention, decision-making, and memory, known collectively as executive functions. Cognition, memory, and IQ are considered complex higher order activities of the brain. Emerging and conflicting evidence in both humans and animals suggest that weed can affect these essential executive functions[255, 256], which are important in normal activity in the brain.

Thinking about things and processing information are known as cognition. It is the mental action of acquiring knowledge, solving problems, and gaining understanding through thought, experience, and the senses[257]. Six types of cognitive processes are attention, perception, memory, use of language, learning, and higher reasoning.

Cognition is malleable, meaning it can change, due in part to neuroplasticity[258]. Neuroplasticity is the ability of the brain to form and reorganize synaptic connections, especially in response to learning or experience or following injury. There is evidence that many things may affect cognitive processes for the better or worse. Some examples of things that may improve cognition in humans for the better include, moderate physical exercise[259], regular fish consumption[260], balance training[261], coffee (interestingly including decaf coffee[262]), and memory training for older adults[263].

It is well known that cognitive decline can be a problem as we age[264]. But, cognition may take a hit at younger ages due to things we do (or don't do), environmental factors we are exposed to, and things we consume. Examples include, alcohol abuse[265], air pollution[266], cardiovascular problems[267], high blood pressure[268], cancer[269], cocaine[270], and cannabis[30, 271, 272].

The effects of marijuana on cognition may be small and are related to how heavy a user you are and how early you start. The good news is that if you stop, those effects appear to be reduced. In a meta-analysis of cannabis and cognitive functioning in adolescents and young adults, in *The Journal of the American Medical Association-Psychiatry,* Scott and colleagues noted, "results indicated a small overall effect size for reduced cognitive functioning associated with frequent or heavy cannabis use", as well as, "continued cannabis use may be associated with small reductions in cognitive functioning, results suggest that cognitive deficits are substantially diminished with abstinence"[273]. Similarly, in a two year study from the University of Minnesota, following 26 heavy cannabis users and 29 non-users ages 18-19 it was found that users "demonstrated weaknesses in verbal learning and memory, spatial working memory, planning, and decision-making relative to non-using demographically matched controls[274].

Cognitive problems are associated with heavy and frequent marijuana use, but tend to resolve with prolonged abstinence[275, 276]. These studies and others[277-283] provide compelling evidence that weed can negatively affect cognition, attention, and other executive functions in adolescents, but stopping cannabis use can mediate those effects.

While the studies described above are about teenagers and young adults, both people in mid-life[284] and older individuals may have cognitive effects due to cannabis as well. In a recent survey[285] of 14,678 people 50 years of age or older in the United States it was stated that "Older marijuana users reported worse cognition compared to never and former users" and "Greater duration and frequency of past use were associated with worse cognition" as well as declines in executive function and attention.

Cannabis, Multiple Sclerosis, and Cognitive Decline

The medicinal use of cannabis to treat the symptoms of multiple sclerosis provides an interesting example of the effects of cannabis on cognition. Cannabis has been shown to help in treating spasticity and pain associated with multiple sclerosis[286], although some studies find little effect[287]. However, there is increasing evidence that cannabis can negatively affect cognition in MS patients. People with MS are a well-monitored group of patients, since they are seen frequently by a neurologist who looks at their changes in brain function over the course of their disease, often using MRI or cognitive tests. These tests often commence before cannabis is prescribed, since the monitoring was initiated due to the diagnosis of MS. Thus, it is possible to compare structural and functional changes in the brains of MS patients before and after cannabis use. A study in 2011[288] from the University of Toronto of cannabis use in multiple sclerosis patients showed that "cannabis users performed significantly more poorly than MS patient nonusers on measures of information processing speed, working memory, executive functions, and visuospatial perception. They were also twice as likely as MS patient nonusers to be classified as globally cognitively impaired." In contrast, a recent report by the same group showed that MS patients using cannabis show significant improvements in memory, processing speed and executive function after 28 days of drug abstinence[289]. Other reports have described cognitive decline and other problems, including depression[290] and earlier age of onset[291], in multiple sclerosis patients that use cannabis for pain management.[292-296] Thus, cannabis induced cognitive decline may be a window on cannabis induced cognitive decline in general.

Memory

There is a lot more to memory[297, 298] than just remembering things. Aspects of memory include explicit memory, implicit memory, prospective memory, semantic memory, episodic memory, short term or working memory, and long term memory. Explicit memory refers to all memories that are consciously available, like where you left your car keys. Implicit memory refers to the use of objects or movements of the body, like how to ride a bicycle. Episodic memory is related to specific events in time, like remembering when you went to the prom. Semantic memory is the ability to recall words, concepts, or numbers.

Prospective memory has to do with remembering something you are planning to do. Most people are familiar with short-term or working memory and long term memory.

The title of a 2018 study[299] from Harvard Medical School that reported on adolescents and young adults that used cannabis regularly, says it clearly: "One Month of Cannabis Abstinence in Adolescents and Young Adults is Associated with Improved Memory".

Figure 4. One Month of Cannabis Abstinence in Adolescents and Young Adults is Associated with Improved Memory.

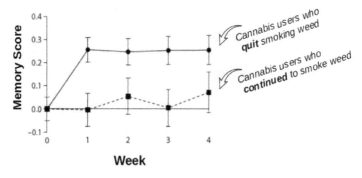

In this study, eighty-eight cannabis users were tested in seven visits over 4 weeks. Sixty two quit cannabis and twenty six continued to smoke. Cognitive tests and urine samples for THC were taken weekly. Improvement in memory was found in the quitters as seen at 1 week, and was maintained for the 4-week testing period. There was no improvement in the cannabis users who continued to smoke. The authors concluded that the study "provides convincing evidence that adolescence and young adults may experience improvements in their ability to learn new information when they stop using cannabis". This corroborated other studies on cannabis and memory[300].

Multiple working memory studies have been performed with functional magnetic resonance imaging (fMRI) in people using cannabis fMRI detects changes in blood flow in the brain when a brain region is activated[301]. With a few exceptions[302, 303], the majority of these studies found altered regional activation in individuals with cannabis during working memory tasks. These included lower brain activation than non-weed users in the right precentral gyrus[304], right hippocampus[305], bilateral middle frontal right dorsolateral prefrontal cortex, and occipital cortex[306]. In addition, greater activation was seen in cannabis users in brain regions including the bilateral superior, middle and inferior frontal gyrus, and over 20 other brain regions[307-311]. There is evidence that alterations in working memory as measured by fMRI may be related to frequency of use of weed[312].

Improvement in Memory?

Can cannabis actually improve cognition or memory in some cases? Interestingly, the study mentioned above from the University of Minnesota demonstrated relative strengths in short term speeded tasks[274]. Other reports describe an improvement in cognitive tasks with cannabis[313-314]. There are also emerging studies in animals that report an improvement in memory[315, 316] in old animals with low dose THC treatment.

Other types of memory has been studied in the context of THC and cannabis such as episodic memory, which is related to memories in time sequence, like what happened three days ago,[317] and episodic foresight[318, 319] which is the ability to project what will happen in the future. A 2012 study of 20 cannabis users versus 20 non-users reported that long-term cannabis users exhibit deficits in prospective memory and executive function[320].

Weed and False Memories

While weed has been shown to affect memory in general, it has also been shown to create false memories[317,321-323].

This may have implications in many aspects of life, but in particular it could have serious ramifications in the context of the questioning of victims and suspects in criminal cases. A significant number of individuals when first encountering law enforcement are under the influence of drugs or alcohol. It has long been known that memory in eyewitness accounts is error prone, but when layering on the influence of weed, it could make matters worse[324, 325]. In 2020, Kloft and colleagues[326] performed a controlled study, using eyewitness and perpetrator scenarios with virtual reality, finding "that cannabis consistently increases susceptibility to false memories". This was for both immediate and delayed recall. The authors state, "the results have implications for police, legal professionals, and policymakers with regard to the treatment of cannabis-intoxicated witnesses and suspects and the validity of their statements."

IQ

What is IQ or Intelligence Quotient? IQ is a score determined from a series of standardized tests that are used to measure intelligence[327]. Does weed affect your IQ? Is the phrase "Let's get stupid" really true? Although the many aspects of IQ are complex, there are multiple studies that report evidence that smoking weed can affect IQ[328-330].

Madeline Meir and colleagues[329], publishing in the *Proceedings of the National Academy of Sciences* in 2012, analyzed the Dunedin Multidisciplinary Health and Development Study, a longitudinal investigation of the health and behavior of a complete birth cohort of consecutive births between April 1, 1972 and March 31, 1973, in Dunedin, New Zealand. This included 1,037 individuals followed from birth to age 38. Neuropsychological testing was done at age 13 before cannabis use started and again at age 38. Cannabis use was determined in interviews at ages 18, 21, 26,

32, and 38 years old. The authors noted, "the most persistent adolescent-onset cannabis users evidenced an average 8-point IQ decline from childhood to adulthood." "Persistent cannabis use over 20 years was associated with neuropsychological decline, and greater decline was evident for more persistent users. This effect was concentrated among adolescent onset cannabis users."

Another study looked at the long term effects of cannabis use while pregnant on the IQ of children. Researchers at the University of Pittsburgh followed 668 offspring[331] from mothers who smoked 1 or more marijuana cigarettes per day. They reported that prenatal use of marijuana by the mother led to children that "had lower intelligence test scores at age 6 than their non-exposed peers." However, findings that cannabis can affect IQ are controversial, with some authors questioning previous analytical approaches or do not find an IQ lowering effect[332, 333].

Cognition, memory and executive function have also been studied extensively in prenatal, adolescent, and adult animal models in the context of cannabis. Animal models using cannabinoids, especially in rats, are very informative since it is possible to test behavior and the brain directly. There are currently over 45 published papers on the effects of THC and cannabis on cognition, memory or executive function in animals. These studies permit the focused use of different doses and specific forms of cannabinoids and a wide range of tests used to measure brain and behavior. These studies generally identify cognitive and memory deficits due to cannabis[220, 334-344], as is found in human studies; although some do not[345, 346].

A study from Indiana University[347] in 2017 showed that chronic adolescent THC treatment of male mice led to long-term cognitive and behavioral dysfunction and impairment of working memory. Interestingly, these effects could be prevented with co-treatment with cannabidiol (CBD). In addition, adult administration of THC did not cause cognitive deficits.

A recent study[348] of prenatal exposure to THC in male rats showed that the formation of aspects of memory was impaired and the development of alcohol-addictive behaviors was promoted. This study expanded upon other observations[349] in animal studies on the negative effects of cannabinoids on offspring of cognition and behavior.

As you think about the effects of cannabis use on cognition, memory, remember the BIG FOUR:
how early, how often, how much, and how strong.

Chapter 7

Cannabis and the Risk of Mental Illness

Psychosis and Cannabis Induced Psychosis; Paranoia; Schizophrenia; The two biggest things about Weed and Schizophrenia; The Chicken or the Egg problem; Depression, Anxiety and Bipolar Disorder, Distress Tolerance and Cannabis.

Psychosis and Cannabis Induced Psychosis

The strongest and most consistent evidence of harm when using marijuana in some people, especially adolescents, is related to psychosis[350, 351] and schizophrenia[16, 179, 352, 353]. Psychosis is a serious psychiatric condition in which someone has problems understanding what is real. Symptoms of psychosis include paranoia, delusions, hallucinations, difficulty concentrating, agitation, and withdrawal from family and friends, among other symptoms[354, 355]. Psychosis can be acute and may resolve for the better, as often occurs in cannabis induced psychosis[356-357], or it may become chronic and may not resolve. There are many causes of psychosis. Psychosis is often a defining characteristic of schizophrenia or bipolar disorder, but also can be caused by some prescription medications, sleep deprivation, or certain neurological disorders. Psychosis is sometimes a feature of alcohol abuse or drug abuse, including weed.

First episode psychosis is the term used when a person experiences psychosis for the very first time and is seen by a physician. When it happens, there are a lot of questions. What behavioral events preceded the psychosis? Is there a family history of psychosis or other psychological disorders? Is there a history of alcohol or drug abuse? Is this going to be a "one off?" Is this cannabis induced psychosis, or might this progress to schizophrenia?

Cannabis induced psychosis[359] is a clinical diagnosis having criteria that distinguishes it from other forms of psychosis, including schizophrenia[356-360]. These criteria include a positive urine test for THC and heavy cannabis use in the last month. Hallucinations and paranoid thoughts are more organized and sequential than in a primary psychosis, symptoms only occur during heavy cannabis use, and symptoms are reduced with abstinence. Typically, symptoms are generally short-lived and total remission often occurs. However, other times the psychosis of cannabis induced psychosis may persist or ultimately be diagnosed as schizophrenia.

In 2019, Marta Di Forti and coworkers reported in the journal *Lancet Psychiatry* that daily use of marijuana and high-potency weed can contribute to developing psychosis. They studied 901 patients with first episode psychosis versus 1237 never user controls at 11 sites in Europe and Brazil. They showed that "daily cannabis use was associated with increased odds of psychotic disorder compared with never users, increasing to nearly five-times increased odds for daily use of high-potency types of cannabis."[361]

Five case studies of first episode psychosis and cannabis are described by Gerlach and coworkers in 2019[362]. These were young adults "between 21 and 26 admitted at the hospital under the clinical appearance of first episode psychosis and a positive THC urine test." On average, they all started marijuana around age 16. They were "hospitalized after a similar pattern of events, following police intervention and emergency medical assistance and arrived disorganized, confused and hostile, with disruptive and unpredictable behavior." They experienced a variety of symptoms including extreme agitation, physical and verbal aggressiveness, confusion, sleep disturbances, disorganization, mood oscillations, paranoid interpretations of reality, and threatening suicide. They were stabilized and treated with medication including antipsychotics and therapy. "In two patients, it was noted that within 12 hours of application of antipsychotic medication, the psychotic substrate fades and rapid recovery occurs. Meanwhile, in the other three, patient's mental state highly oscillated for days followed by gradual improvement of the mental state."[362]

Your chances of having psychosis after smoking weed is a complex brew of 1) weed or extract potency, 2) how often you do it, 3) your metabolism, 4) your age, 5) your sex[363], and 6) your genetic makeup. The risk of psychosis from cannabis use is influenced by common variants of genes, like DRD2 and COMT[364-367] (see Chapter 4).

An important question in weed-induced first episode psychosis is: Will the psychosis persist and take root as schizophrenia or a related long term psychosis? There is emerging evidence that sometimes it does[363,368]. As described by Pearson and Berry in 2020, "this allows for an understanding of the cannabis and psychosis association along something approaching a continuum. Cannabis intoxication becomes Cannabis-Induced Psychotic Disorder once certain severity and duration criteria are met and Cannabis-Induced Psychotic Disorder is heavily associated with future schizophrenia diagnoses"[184].

Paranoia
Paranoia and persecution ideation can be a "one off" as well as a feature of psychosis and schizophrenia. "Paranoid thinking

typically includes persecutory beliefs, or beliefs of conspiracy concerning a perceived threat towards oneself as in,...*Everyone is out to get me*"[369]. Cannabis use has been associated with paranoia and persecution ideation[370, 371]. A study of 1,714 individuals[371] that used cannabis or non-users from around Oxford, UK, found that "the group with a history of cannabis use had significantly higher levels of persecutory ideation compared with the group without a history of cannabis use". Moreover, they state that "there was an approximately three point additional increase in paranoia scores associated with cannabis use in those individuals who had a family history of psychosis." Paranoid ideation is also associated with violence[372]. In the complex mashup of substance abuse, paranoia, and violence, it is not a difficult stretch to suggest that in some individuals cannabis induced paranoia may lead to violence.(see Chapter 10)

Schizophrenia
Schizophrenia is a severe psychiatric disorder characterized by *continuous or relapsing* episodes of psychosis[373] as opposed to a single psychotic event. It is typically not diagnosed at first episode psychosis. A study of over 7,000 individuals in Swe-den concluded, "Schizophrenia following substance-induced psychosis is likely a drug-precipitated disorder in highly vul-nerable individuals, not a syndrome predominantly caused by drug exposure"[374].

THC alters synapse function as well as dopamine based nerve transmission. Evidence suggests that dysfunction of dopamine neurotransmission as well as dysfunction in other brain areas and circuits appears to contribute to the origin of psychotic symptoms in schizophrenia. In addition, disturbances of synaptic function may be the basis of abnormalities of neuronal connectivity[375].

The two biggest things about weed and schizophrenia that can affect you are these:

1. First, really important brain developmental stuff happens at the exact same time that teenagers typically start smoking weed. Brain maturation, vulnerability to schizophrenia, changes in neuronal plasticity due to synaptic pruning[376], and other complex brain changes all happen at the same time. This is the same time when teens are vulnerable to anxiety and depression as well. Compare that to the risk of smoking cigarettes and lung cancer. Teenagers start smoking cigarettes in their teens, but you don't get lung cancer until your 50s, 60s, or 70s. So the threat of cancer is not so real to a teenager. Not so with weed, where you can screw up super critical brain developmental stages as a teenager or young adult[377]. There are no do-overs with brain development.

Figure 5. Age Related Vulnerability to Schizophrenia.

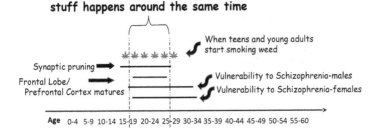

2. The second most important thing for you to know about schizophrenia is: *it can be a life sentence.* You typically get it in late adolescence or early adulthood with around 20% of people having chronic symptoms and disability[375]. Unemployment is extremely high at 80–90%[378]. You often don't pull out of it, and many times it lasts a lifetime.

In a classic study in 1987 of 45,750 young men entering the Swedish army, Andreasson and colleagues[379] showed that men who had used cannabis more than 50 times were six times more likely to experience schizophrenia in the next 15 years than those who had never used it. There is emerging evidence that weed can play a role in the conversion of a less serious condition involving psychosis into actual schizophrenia[380].

The Chicken or the Egg problem

Which comes first, psychosis or use of weed (or both)? There are two longstanding competing theories about which comes first[381-383].

1. The self-medication hypothesis says that people with a predisposition to psychosis, use cannabis in order to alleviate their psychotic symptoms.

2. The damage hypothesis says that using weed exacerbates pre-existing psychotic symptoms or *CAUSES* psychosis or schizophrenia.

It's a complex mashup and complex things don't have simple answers. Here is what we know.

• Cannabis use can predate and predict psychosis in adolescents with no history of previous psychotic disorders[384-387], suggesting a causal relationship.

• Smoking weed can lead to earlier age of onset of psychosis or schizophrenia[388, 389].

• Genetic studies show that starting to use cannabis may be causally associated with the odds of developing psychosis or schizophrenia, *AND* that schizophrenia risk predicts the likelihood of starting cannabis[390].

• The younger you start smoking weed, the greater your chances of developing psychosis[361, 379].

- The continued use of weed makes psychotic symptoms persist after initial diagnosis[386, 391][392].

- The more often you use weed or the stronger the weed you use, the greater chance you have of getting psychosis or schizophrenia[26, 361].

- Cities where daily use of cannabis was common had among the highest adjusted incidence rates of psychotic disorder[361]

- People with gene variants in the genes COMT and AKT1 may be at an increased risk for psychotic disorders in association with cannabinoids. Note that these gene variants do not primarily code for psychosis, they code for more basic brain functions like increased memory, impulsivity, etc., which we all have. These gene variants are *very* common in the population. It is much more likely than not that *you* carry one or more of these gene variants (see Chapter 5).

So, there is very strong scientific evidence from multiple scientific groups worldwide that there is a clear relationship between cannabis use and psychotic disorders, including schizophrenia. There is emerging evidence that this relationship is important in *both* direct causality *and* the effect of cannabis on people with genetic predispositions. In the words of researchers publishing in the medical journal *The Lancet*, "We conclude that there is now sufficient evidence to warn young people that using cannabis could increase their risk of developing a psychotic illness later in life"[351].

Depression, Anxiety and Bipolar Disorder

Depression
The use of cannabis for depression is common in adolescents and adults and the cannabis industry promotes the use of cannabis in depression. However, a major question is: Does regular use and heavy use lead to dependence and increase depression over time? There is clear evidence that over time and

with chronic use, down-regulation of the cannabinoid receptor CB1 in the brain and blunting of the dopamine pathway by cannabis can lead to negative emotionality[140] and anhedonia[393], a reduced ability to experience pleasure.

Depression has been statistically associated with cannabis use[394, 395-397] and the relationship between weed use and depression is complex[398, 399]. Studying the use of weed in depression is complicated because depression is also associated with alcohol and tobacco use, life experiences, and with common genetic variants. However, statistical studies try to separate the effects of weed on depression from other confounding factors. Animal studies are especially valuable in teasing apart the neurobiological complexities of weed on depression.

As described in a 2017 review[400] by Dr. Nora Volkow, the director of the National Institute on Drug Abuse, "the search for a state of mental relaxation and well-being is one of the factors driving the widespread consumption of cannabis. Cannabis enables and enhances the subjective sense of well-being by stimulating the endocannabinoid system (ECS), which plays a key role in modulating the response to stress, reward, and their interactions. However, over time, repeated activation of the ECS by cannabis can trigger neuroadaptations that may impair the sensitivity to stress and reward. This effect, in vulnerable individuals, can lead to addiction and other adverse consequences."

A group of Canadian researchers[397] performed a systematic summary of 14 independent studies on weed and depression that looked at 76,058 individuals. They "found that cannabis use was associated with a modest increased risk for developing depressive disorders. They further found that heavy cannabis use was associated with a stronger, but still moderate, increased risk for developing depression". Their findings "were consistent for cannabis use both in adolescence and in adulthood."

A 2020 study from the Johns Hopkins School of Medicine that studied 14,873 adolescent cannabis users reported[398] that "adolescents with any cannabis use history have significantly higher rates of Major Depressive Disorder[398]", but unexpectedly they found "that heavy users (weekly or greater use) had significantly lower predicted prevalence of lifetime and past year Major Depressive Disorder."

Anxiety

Anxiety is a normal common response to life's stressful situations. It can help us stay alert and be aware of potential danger when necessary. Excessive and continuing anxiety, though, could be a sign of an anxiety-related disorder[401, 402], which may include generalized anxiety disorder, social anxiety disorder, phobias, or separation anxiety disorder[403].

People use cannabis to treat the symptoms of anxiety and there is widespread belief that cannabis and cannabis products help alleviate symptoms of anxiety. Cannabis dispensaries and the cannabis industry promote the use of cannabis for anxiety. The scientific evidence, however, is mixed[399, 404], and there are mixed results in animal models of cannabis and anxiety as well.

Cannabis has the ability to both alleviate the symptoms of anxiety (anxiolytic) and to increase anxiety (anxiogenic) in humans and in animal models[405]. The natural endo-cannabinoid system is intimately involved in the regulation of emotional response[406]. THC tends to be anxiogenic, increasing symptoms of anxiety, while CBD tends to be anxiolytic, reducing symptoms of anxiety[407]. The anxiolytic effect of CBD may "explain why many patients with anxiety disorders use cannabis as a "self-medication" to obtain relief from anxiety symptoms"[405, 408].

There is strong scientific evidence that there is a dose-dependent effect of weed on anxiety. Low dose/short term use of cannabis products may help alleviate symptoms of anxiety while a higher dose and long term use of cannabis can increase anxiety. A study from the University of Chicago in 2017[409] showed that in comparison to a placebo, a low dose of THC significantly reduced self-reported subjective distress in a Social Stress Test, which included the statements; "I feel stressed", "I feel tense", "I feel insecure". However a higher dose of THC "produced small but significant *increases* in anxiety, negative mood and subjective distress". At different doses, neuroimaging data have also demonstrated that THC can both decrease[410] and increase[411] emotional arousal/processing of negative stimuli.

In a 2016 study of anxiety it was shown that "daily or almost daily cannabis use among older adults and Cannabis Use Disorder among younger adults were associated with higher incidence of social anxiety at follow-up"[412] and a 2013 study of adolescents reported that heavy cannabis use in adolescence was in fact associated with higher incidence of any anxiety disorder[413].

It should be clearly stated that when taken in high doses, cannabis can cause intense fear and anxiety, especially in occasional or drug naive users. These may be acute and short-lasting episodes of anxiety, which often resembles a panic attack, in those who are not habitual users[414-416]. Naive users of edibles and concentrates are particularly vulnerable to high dose anxiety and panic outcomes.

The problem with long term cannabis use in anxiety as well as in depression is that long term use can bring habituation or tolerance. As reviewed in 2016[400], in considering cannabis for "anxiety disorders, or depression related stress[417], it should be remembered that repeated use of such medications is bound to down regulate CB1R expression[418, 419]. Such reduction in CB1R expression would result in tolerance to the medication effects[420], thus increasing the risk for depression[421] and perpetuating cannabis dependence[417,422]."

Distress Tolerance and Cannabis

What is distress tolerance? Distress Tolerance (DT) is a concept in psychology that describes how well a person copes with stress. Different people cope with stress differently. It is important in relation to substance use, anxiety, and mood. DT "is a person's ability to manage actual or perceived emotional distress. It also involves being able to make it through an emotional incident without making it worse. People who have low distress tolerance tend to become overwhelmed by stressful situations and may sometimes turn to unhealthy or even destructive ways of coping with these difficult emotions"[423, 424]. Lower distress tolerance (sometimes referred to as distress intolerance) has been shown to be related to more cannabis use in coping with a negative mood[425]. A therapy called Dialectic Behavior Therapy[426], which is related to cognitive behavior therapy has been shown to be effective in improving low distress tolerance in people with substance abuse problems[427].

Bipolar Disorder and Weed

As described by the Mayo Clinic[428], "Bipolar disorder, formerly called manic depression, is a mental health condition that causes extreme mood swings that include emotional highs (mania or hypomania) and lows (depression)...Episodes of mood swings may occur rarely or multiple times a year. While most people will experience some emotional symptoms between episodes, some may not experience any."

Psychosis is the disorder with the strongest connection to weed. However, there is growing evidence that cannabis can influence the course of bipolar disorder. A systematic review of bipolar studies and cannabis in 2015[429] "supported an association between cannabis use and the exacerbation of manic symptoms in those with previously diagnosed bipolar disorder.

Furthermore, a meta-analysis of two studies suggests that cannabis use is associated with an approximately 3-fold increased risk for the new onset of manic symptoms." In addition, they stated cannabis "may worsen the occurrence of manic symptoms in those diagnosed with bipolar disorder, and may also act as a causal risk factor in the incidence of manic symptoms."

In 2007, a prospective study of 3,881 people between 18-64 years of age in the Netherlands concluded, "any use of cannabis at baseline predicted a modest increase in the risk of a first major depression and a stronger increase in the risk of a first bipolar disorder. The risk of 'any mood disorder' was elevated for weekly and almost daily users, but not for less frequent use patterns"[430]. Interestingly, this study did not find any statistically significant associations between cannabis use and anxiety disorders.

Overall, with anxiety and mood disorders taken as a group, a systematic analysis in 2018 of 11,959 individuals[431] concluded, "this review provides consistent evidence that-among individuals living with a baseline PTSD, panic disorder, bipolar disorder, or depressive disorder recent cannabis use was associated with negative symptomatic outcomes over time." "Specifically, the collective findings suggest that individuals using cannabis (ie, any/greater frequency of use in the past 6 months) experienced greater symptom severity and number of symptoms and less occurrence of symptomatic remission and recovery up to five years following baseline assessment relative to the comparison group".

Chapter 8
Pregnancy, Neonatal Issues, and Childhood

Pregnancy and Neonatal Development; The Effects of Prenatal use of Cannabis on Childhood and Adolescence Health; Cannabis Dispensaries are at odds with Health Experts Advice to Pregnant Women; The Lead Toxicity experience versus the Marijuana experience; Unintentional Cannabis ingestion in Young Children.

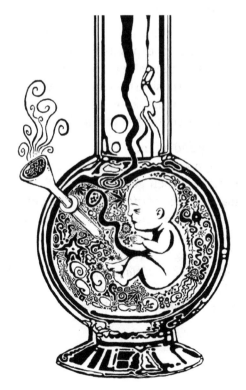

Pregnancy and Neonatal Development

It is sad for me to see a young pregnant woman or a breast-feeding mom smoking weed. That developing baby doesn't have a choice, and that decision to smoke weed could effect that kid for the rest of its life[432]. A study of over 400,000 Australian live births over a 5-year period found that prenatal cannabis exposure increased the risk of neonatal intensive care unit admissions, predominantly for premature birth[433].

THC crosses the placenta into the fetal circulation and can accumulate in the fetus with repeated use of cannabis[442][445]. THC can appear in breastmilk within one hour of consumption and build up in breastmilk with heavy use[434, 435]. THC accumulates in fat. What is one of the major components of breastmilk?...*fat*. Even though cannabis is strongly promoted by marijuana dispensaries for morning sickness and other conditions[436], and use of weed is increasing in pregnant women[437, 438], its use is strongly discouraged by health officials[38, 439-441].

More and more is known about the long-term effects of prenatal or neonatal marijuana exposure on future outcomes in the offspring. There is accumulating evidence that marijuana use in pregnancy increases risk to the fetus and neonate in both the short run (less than 1 year) as well as over the course of childhood and into adolescent development[442-447].

During pregnancy and infancy, THC has been associated with low birth weight, preterm birth, stillbirth or miscarriage, and babies born small for their gestational age[444, 448-456]. In a study, reported in the *American Journal of Perinatology*, of 5,234 women in Washington State, who were tested for the presence of THC[457], the authors found an association between low birth weight and small for gestational age with marijuana use. A large study from Canada, reported in *The Journal of the American Medical Association*, concluded that cannabis use was significantly associated with an increased risk of preterm birth[458]. THC in breastmilk also has been associated with decreased motor development[459] and reduced height[460].

Figure 6. Estimated growth curve and difference infetal weight because of maternal cannabis use[461]

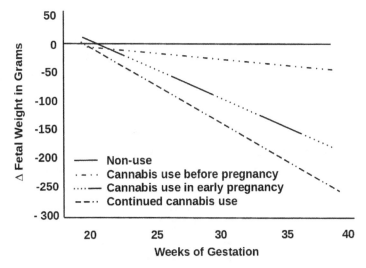

A 2009 report from the University of Amsterdam (figure 6) described reduced fetal weight in grams due to prenatal exposure to cannabis. The authors state that "exposure to potent cannabis in utero may be related to reduced fetal growth and fetal head size, known risk factors for neurodevelopmental and behavioral problems"[461].

The Long Term Effects of Prenatal Cannabis Use on Childhood and Adolescence

There is concern that marijuana use in pregnancy can have long term effects on babies as they grow into children and teenagers. A large Canadian study[462] in 2020 of approximately 500,000 births found a statistical association with prenatal use of cannabis and an increase in autism spectrum disorder. They also found evidence for a smaller increase in intellectual disability, learning disorders, and ADHD, although these were not statistically significant. Further work is needed to establish whether cannabis use is the cause.

Erin Davis and colleagues[434] reviewed the scientific literature for evidence of associations between cannabis use during pregnancy and breastfeeding with altered developmental stage behaviors. These include aggressive behavior and attention deficits at 18 months[462b], and a "significant effect on school age intellectual development" at age 6[462c]. Similar findings on deficits in verbal skills and memory and increases in hyperactivity and impulsivity have been reported[463, 464].

A study from the University of Pittsburgh concludes, "The neurocognitive domains that we have found to be associated with prenatal marijuana exposure by age 10 included depressive symptoms, attention, activity, impulsivity, learning and memory, and IQ"[465]. There are also reports of associations in older children and adolescents due to prenatal use of cannabis by their mothers including changes in behavior and neurocognitive functioning[465,466], decreases in executive function, short-term memory, quantitative and verbal reasoning scores, increases in inattention[463], depressive[467] and anxious symptoms. Likewise, in 18-22 years olds exposed prenatally to cannabis, deficits were found in executive functioning among other factors[468].

This accumulating evidence documents long term effects from smoking weed while pregnant or breastfeeding. I would like to stress that these effects of weed use in pregnancy and breastfeeding don't just affect the baby while you are pregnant, they can play out as the child develops into an adolescent and beyond. Many problems are associated with cannabis use prenatally or while breastfeeding of at least once a week or greater. Also, many of the current published human studies collected data over a time period in the 1970s, 80s, and 90s when THC levels were much lower. Today's weed is much stronger and the potential for health effects are greater.

Are the current human studies definitive? Are they the last word on the subject...No. Are there enough reports to be cautious, concerned, and to think hard about use...Yes. Much more work is needed[469], but there is currently enough evidence to make smart choices. Why put your child at risk? Studies in pregnant animals provides supporting evidence that THC has effects on the developing embryo, its brain, and the placenta[470, 471], as well as having impacts on the offspring[472, 473] on their cognition, behavior[474, 475], and psychological well being[476].

In a recent report published in *Nature Neuroscience*[477], when pregnant rats were exposed to THC, their offspring "exhibit[ed] extensive molecular and synaptic changes in dopaminergic neurons of the ventral tegmental area, including altered excitatory-to-inhibitory balance and switched polarity of long-term synaptic plasticity." They showed that these effects due to prenatal exposure had long term effects in adolescent rats, stating, "the resulting hyperdopaminergic state leads to increased behavioral sensitivity to acute THC exposure during pre-adolescence"[477]. Interestingly, in this model this effect was only found in male offspring and not in females.

This is important. What they are saying is exposure of marijuana to a developing fetus can lead to increased sensitivity to marijuana in the offspring later in pre-adolescence.

These authors speculate that their results, "might manifest in aberrant associative learning and abnormal reward processing, and provides an interpretative framework for clinical studies reporting maladaptive behaviors ranging from affective dysregulation to psychosis and addiction vulnerability in the offspring of mothers using cannabis during pregnancy."[477]

This is one of over 100 scientific studies on the long term effects of the constituents in weed on the offspring of rats and mice during pregnancy. Other animal studies looking at the long term effects on offspring of cannabinoids during pregnancy include their impacts on the endocrine and immune systems[478], glucose homeostasis,[479] movement[480], emotional reactivity[481], cognition[482, 483], and other anomalies[470, 484, 485].

At a molecular, cellular, and developmental level humans brains are very similar to rat brains. If marijuana is altering developing rat brains in highly controlled studies, it is highly likely it is having similar effects on the brains of developing human babies.

Cannabis Dispensaries are at odds with Health Experts Advice to Pregnant Women.

With the increasing evidence of weed's harm during pregnancy, a glaring and dangerous medical inconsistency is that approximately 70% of women in the United States believe that there is "slight or no risk of harm" in using cannabis during pregnancy and approximately 7.5% of expectant moms between the ages of 18 and 25 report using cannabis[486].

To make matters worse, when young women go into a medical cannabis dispensary, more often than not, they are advised to use marijuana for morning sickness and nausea. This is often in the first trimester when the fetus is particularly susceptible to damage from drugs[487, 488]. Dickson and coworkers[436] showed in a statewide cross-sectional study in Colorado that almost 70% of cannabis dispensaries recommended cannabis products to treat nausea in the first trimester. This is exactly the opposite recommendation from doctors and the US Surgeon General. The recommendations from the American College of Obstetricians and Gynecologists advise, "Women reporting marijuana use should be counseled about concerns regarding potential adverse health consequences of continued use during pregnancy"[439]. Likewise, as recommended by the Surgeon General of the United States, "No amount of marijuana use during pregnancy or adolescence is known to be safe. Until and unless more is known about the long-term impact, the safest choice for pregnant women and adolescents is not to use marijuana"[38].

Pregnancy: The Lead Toxicity Experience Versus the Marijuana Experience

Lead ingestion through peeling paint often found in decaying houses in urban areas and lead contamination in public water systems, such as in Flint Michigan, pose a threat to the health of mothers and children, especially minority populations. This is a major health crisis, with public protests, broadly reported in the media, with scathing documentaries.

It has long been known that lead is neurotoxic, and it is particularly harmful to the developing fetus. There is compelling evidence that exposure to lead during pregnancy leads to an increase in the incidence of preterm delivery, birthweight, head circumference[489]. Lead levels in the blood above 10 micrograms per deciliter in children has been shown to reduce IQ by approx-imately 4.25 IQ points as measured at age 38[490]. Here is where direct, carefully controlled toxicity studies in rats are particularly useful. When pregnant rats are exposed to lead, there are changes in the offspring of the growth potential of nerve dendrites in the hippocampus and reduced learning and memory[491].

In addition, breastfeeding human infants are at risk as lead can be passed through breastmilk to a baby. As stated by the American Academy of Pediatrics[492],"low-level lead exposure is a causal risk factor for diminished intellectual and academic abilities, as well as higher rates of neurobehavioral disorders such as hyperactivity and attention deficits, and lower birth weight in children"[493]. The Advisory Committee on Childhood Lead Poisoning Prevention of the Centers for Disease Control and Prevention (CDC) concluded that there is no safe level of lead exposure[494].

Now let's compare the toxicity of lead to weed use in pregnancy; the similarities are striking.

Like lead, THC readily crosses the placenta and enters fetal circulation. THC also accumulates in breastmilk. There is evidence that weed is associated with similar deficits found in lead toxicity in pregnancy including, preterm birth and lower birth weight, as well as being associated with autism[462], intellectual disability, learning disorders and other deficits. Moreover, in a 2012 study on the effect of persistent adolescent cannabis use on IQ, it was reported that "the most persistent adolescent-onset cannabis users evidenced an average 8-point IQ decline from childhood to adulthood"[329]. This finding is controversial and other investigators using a controlled study of twins, publishing in the same journal, attribute this IQ decline to other factors[333]. As with lead toxicity, multiple controlled studies in rat mothers treated with cannabinoids during pregnancy have shown to affect brain function and brain cognition in the offspring later in life[495].

The CDC states that "Marijuana use during pregnancy can be harmful to your baby's health." and that "it is recommended that pregnant women do not use marijuana."[496, 497]. Similarly, the American College of Obstetricians and Gynecologists recommendations[498] regarding marijuana use during pregnancy and lactation are quite clear. They state that, "women reporting marijuana use should be counseled about concerns regarding potential adverse health consequences of continued use during pregnancy." Also, "women who are pregnant or contemplating pregnancy should be encouraged to discontinue marijuana use. There are insufficient data to evaluate the effects of marijuana use on infants during lactation and breastfeeding, and in the absence of such data, marijuana use is discouraged."

Much more work needs to be done. Is there enough data to be cautious? Is there enough data to make wise choices while pregnant? Cannabis dispensaries continue to recommend cannabis for morning sickness in pregnancy. No media attention, no protests, no documentaries? Is it worth the risk to the baby? Think about it. What do you think?

Unintentional Cannabis Ingestion In Young Children

Infants, toddlers, and young kids get into things. They put things into their mouths and eat things they shouldn't. They can inadvertently ingest cannabis or cannabis products, especially resin or haphazardly stored cannabis-containing edibles, like gummies, brownies, or cookies. Other exposures in young children included passive smoke, medical cannabis, beverages, and hemp oil[499]. Common symptoms in children of cannabis exposure are lethargy, loss of body movements, rapid heart rate, dilation of the pupils, and floppy muscles (hypotonia). Serious pediatric consequences can occur including, coma, encephalopathy[500], seizures, and respiratory depression requiring a ventilator[501].

Doctors in Jamaica[500] described a four-year-old boy who was admitted to the emergency room with symptoms of tremors of the hands, blank stare, and inability to speak. He reportedly ingested candy infused with marijuana five hours earlier. He progressively became drowsier and eventually became unresponsive. His urine tested positive for THC. He received treatment with intravenous atropine, oxygen therapy, and maintenance intravenous fluids He recovered after 24 hours of observation.

Colorado began recreational sales of cannabis to the general public on January 1, 2014. Since 2014, the largest increase in reports to the Colorado Regional Poison Center for marijuana exposure has been in children age 0–8 years[502]. Likewise, in a study from France[503], covering the time period 2004-2014[504], there was a 13-fold increase in admissions to a pediatric emergency department for proven cannabis intoxication in children 18 months or younger. This study concluded, "Children are collateral victims of changing trends in cannabis use and a prevailing THC concentration. Intoxicated children are more frequent, are younger, and have intoxications that are more severe."

Chapter 9

Other Very Important Heath-related Stuff

Your Heart and blood vessels; Stroke; Transient Ischemic Attacks; Sleep; Testicular Cancer; Cannabinoid Hyperemesis Syndrome.

Your Heart and Blood Vessels

Cannabinoid receptors that bind THC are not just found in the brain and the nervous system. They are also found on many cells and tissues of the body; in particular on heart muscle, (known as myocardium), aortic smooth muscle, vascular endothelium (the lining of blood vessels), red blood cells, and platelets (the sticky blood cells that form clots)[505]. As in the brain, when THC binds cannabinoid receptors on these tissues, the tissues respond in various ways.

Weed can cause both vasodialation (swelling of the blood vessels), and vasoconstriction[506] (constriction of the blood vessels) resulting in lowered and increased blood pressure respectively. A recent review stated, "Cannabis use results in elevation of heart rate and blood pressure immediately after use, primarily due to sympathetic nervous system stimulation and parasympathetic nervous system inhibition. These effects may precipitate cardiac dysrhythmia"[507].

There are over 200 scientific studies describing cannabis and cardiovascular related health problems. These include papers about acute heart problems[508], cardiovascular disease, stroke, cardiogenic shock[509], arrythmias[510], and heart attack[511-514]. Especially troubling are reports of cardiovascular problems and weed in otherwise healthy young adults[515-517].

While one recent review suggests that marijuana related cardiovascular studies are preliminary and underpowered[518], another recent study analyzing the largest clinical inpatient database in the US, found that during the study period (2010-2014) "major cardiovascular (non-specific chest pain, acute myocardial infarction, congestive heart failure, arrhythmia) and cerebrovascular (stroke and epilepsy) events showed increasing trends among recreational marijuana users."[519]

A 2001 study of 3882 patients[513] showed that the risk of myocardial infarction onset was elevated 4.8 times over baseline in the 60 minutes after marijuana use and rapidly decreased thereafter. Likewise, in 2019 another large study in the medical journal *Anesthesiology*, which studied over 27,000 patients at or around the time of surgery, showed that "an active cannabis use disorder is associated with an increased perioperative risk of myocardial infarction"[520]. In a broad scientific review in 2020 in the medical journal *Circulation*[521], the American Heart Association described multiple adverse effects of Cannabis and made a strongly worded statement saying "the negative health implications of cannabis should be formally and consistently emphasized in policy, including a doubling down on the American Heart Association's commitment to limiting the smoking and vaping of any products and banning cannabis use for youth". Cardiovascular problems with weed may also involve conditions like increases in blood pressure[522], irregular heart beats, and impaired lung function.

Approximately half of adult Americans have some evidence of cardiovascular disease[523] and over 34 million Americans have diabetes[524]. The effects of weed may exacerbate existing conditions related to cardiovascular health such as hypertension, high cholesterol, diabetes, or use of different medications[525]. Baskaren et al. 2019 describe a 60 year old man with hypertension, hyperlipidemia, and diabetes[526] (*how many people does that describe?*) who went to the emergency ward when he had a coronary vasospasm after marijuana ingestion. The authors state that "with the legalization of marijuana in certain states, marijuana-related hospitalizations and ER visits are likely to increase."

Jack Herer—The Emperor of Hemp

Jack Herer (1939-2010)[527] was a pro-cannabis and hemp activist and founded the organization Help End Marijuana Prohibition (HEMP). He wrote the non-fiction book, *The Emperor has no Clothes,* about cannabis, and hemp for industrial purposes. He was sometimes called "The Emperor of Hemp". He ran for President of the United States twice as the Grassroots Party candidate. Jack Herer had his first heart attack and a major stroke at the age of 61. He had his second heart attack 9 years later at the Hempstalk Festival in Portland, Oregon. He died seven months later in Eugene, Oregon from complications related to the heart attacks and stroke. The sativa-dominant strain of cannabis, *Jack Herer,* is named in his honor. Was weed related to his multiple heart attacks or stroke? Hard to say, on one hand there is no direct evidence it did. On the other hand...weed is associated with heart attacks and stroke. Overweight guy in his sixties, smoked a lot of weed... something to think about.

Arrhythmias

Arrhythmias are irregular heart beats[528], in which your heart beats too quickly, too slowly, or in an irregular pattern. In a recent study of the admissions at over 4,000 US hospitals, researchers investigated the prevalence of cardiac arrhythmias in teenage cannabis users[529]. They identified multiple symptoms related to arrhythmias including, ventricular fibrillation, heart palpitation, QT syndrome, and atrial flutter. These were teenagers age 13 to 19. While not very frequent (36-513 in 100,000), it happens. Another report[530], described a 19 year old who experienced three episodes of near complete loss of consciousness in the hours prior to seeing a doctor. He was found to have a "complete heart block" and was treated. He was "advised to quit using cannabis". Follow up testing with ECG monitoring, "after cessation of cannabis use, showed normal sinus rhythm without atrioventricular block."

Stroke
Stroke is caused by blockage in a blood vessel that restricts blood flow to the brain, causing damage to brain tissue. It is the 5th highest cause of death and a leading cause of disability in the US[531]. As reported in 2019[532], "a 37 year old male with no significant medical history was brought in by his father with complaints of worsening mental status and functional decline". He told the doctors he had been smoking 3 grams of weed every day since he was 12 years old. He was diagnosed as having acute and chronic ischemic stroke in his brain. After eight days of hospitalization and anti-coagulation therapy he was discharged to an inpatient rehabilitation unit.

A recently published epidemiological study analyzing data from the Centers for Disease Control and Prevention concluded that "there may be a significantly higher odds of stroke in young marijuana users (18-44 years) as compared to non-users with even greater odds among frequent users (>10 days/month)"[517]. Another recent large epidemiological study of over 3 million hospitalizations of all kinds from 2007-2014 "identified rising trends and higher risk (16% higher of overall young-onset stroke, 41% higher of acute ischemic stroke) of stroke-related hospitalizations and worse outcomes among cannabis users aged 18-49 years"[533].

Transient Ischemic Attacks—TIAs

A Transient Ischemic Attack is often referred to as a mini-stroke. Like strokes, they are caused by a disruption in blood flow to the brain, or cerebral blood flow and may result in a brief episode of neurological dysfunction[534, 535].

The effects are generally temporary and may include weakness or numbness on one side of the body, dimming or loss of vision, difficulty speaking or understanding language, slurred speech, and confusion. They may be a warning sign of a future stroke. A 2016 study of over 7,000 people in the general population in Australia found that those who used cannabis weekly or more often had 3.3 times the rate of stroke/TIA than those that did not use cannabis. There was no increase in those who used cannabis less often[536].

Dr. Ann M. Mousak describes a 26-year-old male, who was a heavy cannabis smoker, who appeared with partial paralysis on the right side of the body (hemiparesis) and speech difficulties (aphasia) 3 hours after smoking a large amount of cannabis. The patient's symptoms lasted 24 h. The patient reported cannabis abuse since the age of 16. No other drug abuse was recorded except for light tobacco smoking. Transient amnesia, episodes of gait disequilibrium and confusion was found. Dr. Mousak also described two similar cases involving TIAs shortly after smoking large amounts of cannabis. "They did not have any risk factors for small-vessel disease. The meticulous and extensive examinations revealed only cannabis as the possible causative agent"[537].

Sleep

"The only time I have problems is when I sleep."

—*Tupac Shakur*

Sleep is essential for many aspects of good health and wellbeing. Dysfunctional sleep can lead to a host of physical and psychological problems. The natural endocannabinoid system in the brain is important in helping you sleep. The molecules anandamide and 2-AG bind the cannabinoid receptor CB1 on neurons in the brain and help regulate sleep[136]. Experimental administration of anandamide in animals increases rapid eye movement (REM) sleep and non-REM sleep[538, 539].

Cannabis has been used to induce sleep for centuries. In 1843 John Clendinning, M.D., a physician to the St. Marylebone Infirmary, London, U.K., described a case where..."a medical man of forty-four...at bed-time, being in good health, took 12 minims of Squire's tincture of Indian hemp, which are equivalent to 1 grain of the extract. In a few minutes he perceived that slight sense of confusion and fullness in the head...in half an hour or thereabout fell into a slumber which lasted, uninterruptedly, for about six hours...this gentleman rarely sleeps more than three or four hours consecutively"[540].

Insomnia and other sleep problems are one of the main reasons people use medicinal cannabis. Although, the cannabis industry strongly promotes cannabis for sleep problems, there is mixed scientific evidence[542, 543] that cannabinoids have a long term benefit on sleep[99]. While some studies show a reduction in sleep onset latency[543], how quickly you fall to sleep, others do not replicate that finding. A small short term study in 2020 of middle-aged and older adults reported preliminary results indicating cannabis use may have a positive effect on sleep duration[544]. There is preliminary evidence in both animal studies[545] and in people with medical conditions that disrupt their sleep (such as sleep apnea[546], chronic pain[547], anxiety[548], restless leg syndrome[549], or nightmares in PTSD[550]) that cannabinoids may help the primary health issue, thus allowing for better sleep. Most controlled clinical trials that look at sleep and cannabinoids use pharmaceutical grade cannabinoids (e.g., Dronabinol, Sativex, and Epidiolex) rather than recreational marijuana.

Overall, an emerging pattern from human sleep studies may be related to the bi-phasic effects of THC or *Short term use-ok; Long term use-bad* (see Chapter 3). As reviewed by Babson and coworkers in 2017, early studies suggest that cannabis may have a short-term benefit on sleep, particularly in reducing the time to fall asleep. But long term, chronic use of cannabis may lead to habituation to these sleep-inducing effects. Habituation is a decrease in response to a stimulus after repeated use. These investigators state, "Long-term use could have a negative impact on sleep in two primary ways. First, individuals may find themselves in a vicious cycle of using cannabis to manage sleep, but ultimately habituating to the effects. This makes people use more cannabis in order to obtain the desired effect, resulting in problematic patterns of use. Second, sleep disturbances are the hallmark of cannabis withdrawal and may serve to maintain use and predict relapse"[542].

People who regularly use cannabis, especially heavy users, exhibit sleep disruption[551], particularly during withdrawal from cannabis use. Sleep disturbance is a frequent complaint of about 76% of daily cannabis users who abruptly discontinue their cannabis use[552]. Symptoms reported include sleep difficulties such as strange dreams, insomnia, and poor sleep quality[553]. Abrupt discontinuation of daily, or near daily cannabis use may lead to abstinence-induced insomnia[551].

Adolescents and young adults are particularly at risk for sleep problems. In an analysis of 1,125 students aged 17 to 24 years from an urban Midwestern university, over 60% were categorized as poor-quality sleepers[554]. A study published in the *Journal of American College Health* in 2019 of 354 college students[555] found that using marijuana to aid in sleep was "associated with worse sleep efficiency. Sleep problems related to daytime dysfunction was found to predict increased marijuana use in the past month, and more problematic use in the past month and past year".

Sleep is complex and so are sleep studies. Alcohol use, nicotine co-use, and other concurrent medical issues can also disrupt sleep and may cloud the direct effect of cannabis on sleep. These, and other issues complicate self-reports of the effect of subjective effects of Cannabis on sleep. More well controlled clinical trials on Cannabis and cannabinoids and sleep are needed.

Testicular Cancer

Cancer...never a welcome word. Testicular cancer is relatively rare, accounting for less than 2% of male cancers; however, it is the most common malignant neoplasm occurring in young men, ages 15-44[556].

The endocannabinoid system is important in sperm biology and fertility[557]. Marijuana has been shown to alter sperm numbers, testicular function, and hormone levels[558] in both humans and animals, although this data is sometimes conflicting. In the context of these complex effects on testicular biology, there is emerging evidence that marijuana can increase the risk for testicular cancer in heavy users[556, 559]. In a 42 year follow-up of over 49,000 Swedish men[560] between 1970 and 2011, the risk of testicular cancer increased by 2.5-fold if you had smoked weed greater than 50 times in your lifetime. Similarly, a systematic review of cancer and marijuana in 2019 published in the *Journal of the American Medical Association-Network Open* reported that more than 10 years of marijuana use was associated with testicular cancer[561]. Interestingly, they also found that evidence of the association between marijuana use and incident lung cancer was insufficient due to a lack of high quality data. Lower usage of weed was not associated with cancer.

Cannabinoid Hyperemesis Syndrome

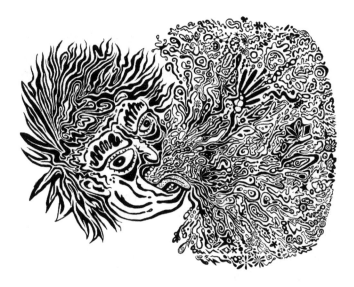

Everyone knows smoking weed can give you the munchies, but did you know it can also give you the serious pukes?

Sometimes people use cannabis for nausea without knowing heavy use can *cause* nausea or make it worse. Emesis is the medical term for vomiting. Hyperemesis is persistent severe vomiting leading to weight loss and dehydration. Cannabinoid Hyperemesis Syndrome[562][563-566] is a rare condition of cyclical vomiting and nausea found occasionally in heavy marijuana users; weekly or daily use[567]. In a 2018 study[568] from the New York University School of Medicine, patients that entered the hospital for multiple reasons were asked if they smoked weed 20 or more days per month. They then were evaluated on a ten point scale for nausea and vomiting. Over thirty two percent met the criteria for having experienced Cannabinoid Hyper-emesis Syndrome.

Symptoms may include; ongoing nausea, repeated episodes of vomiting, belly pain, decreased food intake, weight loss, and dehydration[569]. These symptoms may continue until the person completely stops using marijuana. Often hot showers are taken, sometimes compulsively[570], to help with the nausea. In some cases hospitalization may be required and fatalities have been reported. It is a paradox that cannabis can both help the symptoms of nausea and cause nausea. One theory[570, 571] is that "chronic, heavy cannabis use may cause cannabinoid receptors in the gut to override the effect of cannabinoid receptor stimulation in the brain, thereby leading to paradoxical hyperemesis"[572].

A 38 year old male showed up at the emergency ward with acute nausea, vomiting and unrelenting gastric pain for 5 days[572]. He reported vomiting that occurred 10–12 times per day. He had vomiting episodes for the past 20 years, occurring 3–4 times a month, lasting for an average of 7 days. He reported smoking marijuana regularly for the past 20 years, smoking an average of 5–6 joints per day. The patient was examined for any medical complications and treated with saline, anti-nausea medications and a heartburn medication for gastritis. The patient was advised to stop the use of marijuana completely to stop these recurring symptoms.

Chapter 10
Societal Related Stuff

Educational Achievement; Motivation; Employment and Jobs; Conflating Legalization issues with Health Issues; Driving; Violence; Suicide; and PTSD.

Educational Achievement

There is increasing and compelling scientific evidence that starting weed at an early age and smoking a lot of weed for a long time is associated with lower educational and job achievement[573,574,574b,575]. As noted in a review in *JAMA Psychiatry* by Nora Volkow M.D., the director of the National Institute on Drug Abuse, "there is evidence that long-term heavy cannabis use is associated with educational underachievement and impaired motivation"[16][576-578]. This association of heavy use of weed with educational achievement is complex. There may be direct effects on brain cognition, motivation[573-579], or on social aspects that affect behavior and personal relationships. A large study in Australia and New Zealand, found that those who were daily users of cannabis before age 17 years had clear reductions in the odds of high school completion and degree attainment[580], as well as an increase in other bad outcomes including later cannabis dependence[580], use of other illicit drugs, and suicide attempts[581]. A similar study in Canada in 2018 found significant differences in educational attainment[78]. Both increasing users and chronic users reported lower educational attainment and occupational prestige.

Different trajectories of use of weed in adolescence have been shown to have different educational outcomes when seen at the population level. In a study of 5,322 people from age 13-23, 5 trajectories of weed use were identified; *abstainers, occasional light users, stable light users, steady increasers, and early high users.* "Abstainers consistently had the most favorable (behavioral, socioeconomic, and health outcomes at age 29), whereas early high users consistently had the least favorable outcomes."[582]

In a similar study in 2015 of 808 individuals from ages 14 through 30, Marina Epstein and her colleagues at the University of Washington reported that a pattern of adolescent, late-onset or chronic use of weed resulted in worse educational and economic outcomes than did non-users[583].

Like education, obtaining and holding a job may be negatively affected by starting weed early in adolescence and with heavy use. Education and employment are of course highly related. There is conflicting evidence on the relation between cannabis use and job outcomes. Some studies show no or weak effects on employment using certain statistical approaches[584] while other studies show specific effects on employment[10, 585-587], particularly for heavy users of weed. French researchers studying 18,879 workers aged 18–69 years found that cannabis (as well as alcohol and tobacco) use was positively associated with job loss at one-year after adjusting for age, gender, depressive symptoms, and self-rated health[588]. There are also reports that weed can have a positive effect on wages in the short run[589]. What's up with that?

Does weed cause a lack of motivation or an increase in apathy, which plays out in many different directions like school or jobs[593]? It's hard to say. It is very difficult to statistically separate motivation from other confounders related to amotivation such as depression, personality differences, and alcohol and other substance use. These multiple factors tend to act together.

Some researchers find no evidence of amotivation and weed. However, other researchers have shown statistically significant correlations with cannabis use and amotivation[590] and apathy[152, 577-579], possibly in the context of Dopamine dysfunction. Interestingly, one study showed "cannabis without CBD led to an overall reduction in motivation[594]. Cannabis with CBD did not appear to reduce this effect but did moderate THC's effects"[594].

Motivation, Amotivation and White Russians

Motivation (moh-tuh-vey-shuhn) Definition: the state or condition of being motivated or having a strong reason to act or accomplish something. As opposed to Amotivation[590], or the lack of motivation.

The classic stoner, Jeffrey "The Dude" Lebowski, from the movie "The Big Lebowski"[591], slacker, bowler, and White Russian enthusiast...could be said to be in a chronic state of Amotivation...but in his words, "Yeah, well, you know, that's just, like, your opinion, man."–The Dude[592]

Conflating Decriminalization/Legalization of Cannabis and Health related issues

Conflate /kən'flāt/ -to combine two or more ideas, etc. into one.

A major factor driving the decriminalization and legalization movements of cannabis is the failure of the war on drugs, which has been not only ineffective, but has resulted in untold societal effects and harmful effects on individual lives due to falling into the criminal justice system and incarceration. Often public discussion driving cannabis legislation centers on incarceration and decriminalization issues, while ignoring important health related issues. Also, central to any discussion of legalization is a potential increase in revenue from taxing cannabis sales. However, the push to change the legal aspects of cannabis for whatever reason does not mean that the health issues related to cannabis use have changed. Those issues should not be conflated.

Driving

The THC in weed is a psychoactive agent. It messes with your judgment, thinking, attention, psychomotor skills, as well as your time and space perception[595, 596]. And yes, it interferes with your ability to drive, both while you are high and in chronic long time users. Ironically, with the legalization of recreational marijuana, the public perception of safety and driving may become confused[597], with many people thinking that it is safe to drive after using marijuana. A driving simulator study in California reported that "Chronic marijuana users had slower reaction times, deviated less in speed, and had difficulty matching a lead vehicle's speed compared to nonusers"[598]. In a study of car crashes, Cook and coworkers looked at 24 American cities between 2010 and 2017 and showed a "13% increase in fatal crashes involving 15 to 24-year-old male drivers following marijuana decriminalization...This effect was immediate and strongest on weekend nights."[599]. Interestingly, they did not find an increase in crashes in females and older males. They also saw a decrease in crashes related to the introduction of Medical Marijuana laws which require consumption at home. This increase in marijuana related crashes has also been found in different countries including Australia[600], Uruguay[601], and Canada[602]. In a systematic review of 19 scientific publication databases, it was concluded that, "acute cannabis consumption is associated with an increased risk of a motor vehicle crash, especially for fatal collisions"[603]. Whatever way you look at it, smoking weed and driving can be a fatal mix. That's not to mention the mixing of alcohol, weed, and driving, which of course happens all the time. What teenage party does not have both alcohol and weed?

Violence, Suicide, and PTSD

Violence has been associated with marijuana use in population studies from around the globe[604-608]: including in Canada[605], Scandinavia[608], remote aboriginal communities in Australia[609], England[610], Switzerland[611], and the United States[612, 613]. This is often in the context of impulsivity, psychosis or mental illness. These are small but statistically significant associations in the overall population, but at an individual level, the results can be tragic.

Weed can induce psychosis in some individuals, psychosis can lead to violence in some people. Not in everybody, not in many people, but in a few troubled individuals. In his excellent book "Tell Your Children" Alex Berenson describes the history, science and individual stories of psychotic breaks after using marijuana leading to violence, often out of nowhere. The stories are painfully sad and heartbreaking[614, 615].

In a review of incidents of heavy marijuana use and violence, Norman Miller and colleagues describe[604] recent high profile cases of extreme violence including; Nikolas Cruz in 2018 at the Marjory Stoneman Douglas High School in Parkland, Florida; Dylan Roof in 2015 at Emanuel AME church in Charleston, South Carolina; Devin Patrick Kelley in 2017 at the First Baptist Church in Sutherland Springs, Texas, and Jared Loughner in 2011 at US Representative Gabrielle Giffords's political event in Tucson, Arizona. All of these young men were heavy marijuana users from a young age, and suffered from paranoia and mental illness, including hearing voices.

Cannabis and violence is not just about high profile cases. Weed has been positively associated with dating violence and intimate partner violence. Johnson and colleagues showed that marijuana use is associated with physical dating violence in adolescents as both the victim and the perpetrator[616]. Similarly, Shorey and coworkers[617] demonstrated that marijuana is associated with intimate partner violence perpetration among men arrested for domestic violence.

The role of weed in violence is very complex and much more study is needed. Does weed induce violence on its own? Is it a trigger? Does it happen in many people? Almost certainly not for all of these, but in the witches brew of long term use, strong THC content, genetic risk, increasing paranoia and mental illness, things can go horribly wrong in some individuals.

Suicide

Suicide is tragic violence to oneself. Factors that contribute to suicide, suicide attempts, and suicide ideation[618] (thoughts about suicide) are many and complex[619]. Among those factors are depression, psychosis, bipolar disorder and other mental health issues; being between the ages of 15 and 24 years or over age 60, a family history of suicide, and substance abuse, including weed[620, 394, 621, 622].

In a recent study of over 86,000 adolescents aged 12–15 years from 21 low- and middle-income countries, Carvalho and coworkers[623] found that cannabis use in the past 30 days was associated with a 2.03 times higher odds for suicide attempts. This was after adjustment for other complicating factors including alcohol consumption, amphetamine use, smoking, and anxiety-induced insomnia. This is a statistical association. The authors clearly state that further work needs to be done to show causality.

In a meta-analysis of multiple studies from different populations and using different statistical methods on suicide and cannabis use from 1990-2015[624], it was found that "The evidence tends to support that chronic cannabis use can predict suicidality". However, that finding was tempered by the variation introduced by different study parameters.

Tom King Forcade

Tom King Forcade[625 626], was a drug smuggler, cannabis activist, and journalist. He was a colorful character in the early counterculture days of the marijuana movement in the United States. He ran the Underground Press Syndicate and founded the magazine High Times in 1974 which promotes the legalization and use of weed. By 1977 High Times was selling as many copies an issue as Rolling Stone and National Lampoon. Forcade gained notoriety in 1970 by hitting Chairman Otto Larsen in the face with a cream pie during the President's Commission on Obscenity and Pornography. Forcade was increasingly plagued by depression and paranoia. He committed suicide at the age of 33, shooting himself in the head on November 17, 1978[625, 626].

Post Traumatic Stress Disorder

Cannabis is commonly discussed in the general public as a therapeutic approach in Post Traumatic Stress Disorder (PTSD), especially with respect to returning veterans. Although using weed to alleviate the symptoms of PTSD is controversial[627], in fact, there is little scientific evidence that smoking weed helps aspects of PTSD, although more study is needed. A recent study from University College London concluded that "The clinical effectiveness of cannabinoids for the treatment of PTSD remains largely hypothetical; there is insufficient and poor-quality evidence of the effectiveness of cannabinoids for PTSD."[628]

There is growing evidence that marijuana may make symptoms of PTSD *worse*, including Cannabis Use Disorder and suicide.[629, 630] In a 2015 study from Yale University, the title spells it out "Marijuana use is associated with worse outcomes in symptom severity and violent behavior in patients with posttraumatic stress disorder". They studied 2,276 veterans with PTSD. When compared to veterans who had never used weed, stopping weed improved PTSD symptoms while starting weed increased PTSD symptoms.[631]

Marujuana use and PTSD have both been associated with abnormalities in brain white matter. In a recent brain imaging analysis of the white matter of PTSD patients that either used or did not use weed, marijuana did not improve brain white matter abnormalities.[632]

In a 2019 study of cannabis dependence and post-deployment suicide attempts in Iraq/Afghanistan-era veterans, Kelsie Adkisson, and colleagues[633] from the Veterans Administration Mid-Atlantic Mental Illness Research, Education, and Clinical Center, found that lifetime cannabis dependence is associated with post-deployment suicide attempts among veterans.

Conclusion

Science is a constantly flowing river. Evidence accumulates every day. We are always in a position of knowing many things, but always wanting to know more. At the same time, we as individuals are faced with having to make health and life decisions on any given day sometimes using incomplete and imperfect information. What do we do today with what we know right now? My guess is that most thoughtful people make important life decisions as best they can in the face of uncertainty. They weigh the best information currently available and decide which path to take.

What I have described in this book is the peer reviewed scientific evidence that Cannabis and Cannabis products can harm your health, the health of your kids, your friends, and your neighbors. I have only scratched the surface of the more than 35,000 peer reviewed scientific publications on Marijuana. Much of this work is ongoing and more work is always needed, but there is clearly an overwhelming amount of data that documents Cannabis associated harm.

While many people have no problems associated with Cannabis, many do. Especially vulnerable are developing babies, adolescents and young adults, people with underlying medical conditions, and people with a family history of substance abuse or common mental and psychological conditions, such as anxiety, depression, or bipolar disorder. That's a lot of people.

By far, most of the health problems associated with Cannabis are related to: How early you start, How often you use it, How much you consume, and How strong it is. Of course the simplest way to avoid these health problems is to not use cannabis or cannabis products.

How might cannabis use affect you in the sort term and in the long term? How does it affect your kids and the people around you? I have introduced you to the current state of scientific evidence. Think on these things. Make your own decisions. May your own path lead to good health, happiness, and well being.

Remembering Mark

Mark was my older brother, by 14 months. My only sibling. He was a nice guy, very shy, sometimes funny, tall and very skinny as a teenager. At 19 he looked like James Taylor. He wore a top hat, played acoustic guitar. His nickname as a teenager was "Skel" for Skele-teen. Hey Skel, what's up?

He was quite the stoner in high school. He would hide his weed in the heating vents in the floor of his room. Our parents always found it, but he would still hide it there. He had a subscription to "*High Times*". He painted his bedroom black. Later in life, I asked him, "Mark. Did you smoke a lot of weed in high school?". He said..."no...no...I smoked a lot of Hash!"

After graduating from high school, he took some classes at a local community college and worked at various jobs for a short while. Worked in a restaurant at the beach one summer. Around age 18 or 19 he started sleeping all day and acting and talking erratically. Our parents got him counseling, but it didn't help. It got worse. Then he started acting really weird and was picked up by the local police and spent a night in the local slammer.

He was diagnosed as schizophrenic around age 21. He would go off and on his medication. When he was home he would throw his medication out the window, he said he wanted to grow "Mellaril trees". He climbed out a window and disappeared one day. After about three weeks he was arrested over 2,000 miles away in eastern Nevada. A friend and I drove an old pickup truck to get him and brought him home where he first entered a psychiatric hospital. He spent time in 5 or 6 psychiatric hospitals, finally spending 5 years in Maryland's maximum security forensic psychiatric hospital. That was quite grim. When he got out of that hospital he was a changed person, very passive with a flat affect.

He moved to a very nice town on the Chesapeake bay close to my parents, went to a day center and lived in group homes for about 10 years. He then got his own subsidized apartment and lived on disability until the age of 65, when he had a heart attack and passed away. In that town, he had a wonderful dedicated network of support from health professionals and caring people for which I will be eternally grateful.

After he got sick, he never held a job, never had a girlfriend, never played guitar again, never read a book. He was a chronic schizophrenic, confused for 45 years. Do I know that weed caused his schizophrenia? No. What I do know is that it sure as hell didn't help. Take care Skel.

About the Author

Kevin G. Becker received a Ph.D. from the Johns Hopkins University School of Medicine in 1989 in Molecular Biology and Genetics. He spent 30 years as a scientist in the Intramural Research Program at the U.S. National Institutes of Health. This included postdoctoral fellowships at the National Institutes of Child Health and Human Development, Neurological Diseases and Stroke, and The National Human Genome Research Institute. He was a Staff Scientist at the National Institute on Aging for over 20 years. He has published on a broad range of topics including aging, autoimmune disease including multiple sclerosis, autism, bioinformatics, gene expression, genetics, immunity, metabolism and neuroscience. At the NIA he often collaborated with investigators from the National Institute on Drug Abuse. He is an author or co-author on over 300 peer reviewed scientific publications.

About the Illustrator

Ned Hopkins is an artist and illustrator from Baltimore, Maryland. A graduate of the Savannah College of Art and Design, his work spans both digital and traditional mediums. Find more of his drawings and paintings at http://nedhopkinsart.com/

Michael Zierler
Science editor
Ulster County, New York
https://www.linkedin.com/in/michael-zierler-science-editor/

Wayne Kehoe
Graphic designer and typographer
http://www.waynekehoe.com | info@waynekehoe.com

Glossary and Useful Definitions

Scientific review paper—a scientific paper that discusses multiple published papers on the same or similar topics, with the aim of distilling or summarizing the current findings found in those papers. Sometimes the summary consolidates the findings, however sometimes the summary reveals that there is no consensus on the topic. Typically they come in different styles such as; narrative review, meta-analysis, or systematic review.

Scientific research study—a controlled analysis of a medical or scientific topic which records, collects, analyzes, and summarizes data. These come in different types including; experimental study, observational study (where you only observe and record data), interventional study (where you intervene or give drugs or compounds), association study (which is primarily statistically based), longitudinal study (which takes place over a long period of time), and cross sectional study (which analyzes data acquired all at one time).

Bi-phasic response—two separate and distinct responses that are separated in time.

SNPs Single Nucleotide Polymorphism—a nucleotide position in the DNA that is variable, being one of either A, T, C, or G.

Gene—a gene is a basic unit of heredity and a sequence of nucleotides in DNA, that encodes RNA for the synthesis of a gene product, either RNA or protein.

Gene variant—a specific region of the gene which differs between two individuals.

Dopaminergic—releasing or involving dopamine as a neurotransmitter. hyperdopaminergic – an excessive dopaminergic response and hypodopaminergic – significantly reduced levels of dopamine as opposed to normal levels.

Cognition—the mental action or process of acquiring knowledge and understanding through thought, experience, and the senses.

Epigenetics—epigenetics is the study of heritable phenotype changes that do not involve alterations in the DNA sequence.

Cardiac arrhythmia or dysrhythmia —cardiac dysrhythmias are problems with the rate or rhythm of your heartbeat caused by changes in your heart's normal sequence of electri-cal impulses.

Poly Substance Use—the consumption of multiple legal or ille-gal substances over a defined period or simultaneously. These may include alcohol, cannabis, nicotine including vaping nico-tine, opioids, cocaine, methamphetamine, or other substances.

Genus species versus strain—The official systematic Genus of marijuana is *Cannabis*. Two species of Cannabis are *sativa* and *indica*. The word strain has no official botanical meaning and is used for varieties of *Cannabis sativa* or *Cannabis indica* which have been bred to strengthen different traits including THC or CBD content, growing properties, or different terpenes.

Cannabinoid—A chemical found in cannabis.

Terpenes—Organic compounds that provide aroma and flavor in cannabis and other plants.

Edibles—a food infused with cannabinoids. When marijuana is ingested, cannabinoids enter the bloodstream through the digestive system, which increases potency, delays the onset of effects and may lengthen the intoxicating effects.

Dabbing or Dabs—the use of cannabis concentrate, often from butane hash oil, often used through a vaporizer.

Shatter—a brittle, glass-like concentrated cannabis extract with a tendency to snap when handled.

Wax—a cannabis concentrate named for its appearance and texture. It has an opaque, thick, malleable, wax-like consistency

To go directly to the publications for many of the following references:

Go to the PubMed web-site:
https://www.ncbi.nlm.nih.gov/pubmed and type just the PMID number in the PubMed search box and hit enter.

Or go to the PubMed Central web-site:
https://www.ncbi.nlm.nih.gov/pmc/
and type just the PMC number in the search box and hit enter.

You can click through directly to most of the abstracts, papers or websites in the References from:
Whoa Dude Online References https://whoadude-the-book.com/references

References

Chapter 2: Getting Your Bearings: Refs. 1-10
Different Levels of Scientific Evidence; Statistical Associations versus Causality; Multiple Studies from Different Research Groups; Older Data or Newer Data In the World of Weed; PubMed and PubMed Central;

Ten Excellent Free Reviews

1. Macdonald K. and Pappas K.. WHY NOT POT? A Review of the Brain based Risks of Cannabis. Innovations in Clinical Neuroscience 2016;13{3-4}:13-22. PubMed PMID_27354924_PubMed Central PMC4911936. FREE

2. Volkow, N. et. al. Adverse Health Effects of Marijuana Use. New England Journal of Medicine. 2014 Jun 5; 370{23}: 2219-2227. PubMed PMID24897085_PubMed Central PMC4827335. FREE

3. Zehra A. et al. 2018 Cannabis Addiction and the Brain: a Review Journal of Neuroimmune Pharmacology 2018; 13{4}: 438-452. PubMed PMID29556883_PubMed Central PMC6223748. FREE

4. Memedovich KA, et al. The adverse health effects and harms related to marijuana use: an overview review CMAJ Open 2018. PubMed PMID30115639_PubMed Central PMC6182105. FREE

5. Murray, R.M. et al. Traditional marijuana, high-potency cannabis and synthetic cannabinoids: increasing risk for psychosis World Psychiatry. 2016 Oct; 15{3}:

195–204. PubMed PMID27717258_ PubMed Central PMC5032490. FREE

6. Grant C and Belanger . Cannabis and Canada's Children and Youth. Paediatr Child Health 2017 May;22{2}:98-102. PubMed PMID29480902_ PubMed Central PMC5804770. FREE

7. De Aquino JP, Sherif M, Radhakrishnan R, Cahill JD, Ranganathan M, D'Souza DC. The Psychiatric Consequences of Cannabinoids. Clin Ther. 2018 Sep;40{9}:1448-1456 PubMed PMID29678279. FREE

8. Hasin DS US Epidemiology of Cannabis Use and Associated Problems. Neuropsychopharmacology. 2018 Jan; 43{1}: 195–212. PubMed PMID28853439_PubMed Central PMC5719106. FREE

9. Archie S.R. and Cucullo L. Front Pharmacol. Harmful Effects of Smoking Cannabis: A Cerebrovascular and Neurological Perspective. 2019; 10: 1481. PubMed PMID31920665_ PubMed Central PMC6915047. FREE

10. Beverly HK, Castro Y, Opara I. Age of First Marijuana Use and Its Impact on Education Attainment and Employment Status. J Drug Issues. PubMed PMID31341332_PubMed Central PMC6655417. FREE

Chapter 3: Things to know about weed: Refs. 11-42
The Big 4-How early, How often, How much, How strong; Low Dose /High Dose-Short Term /Long Term use; People are different; This is not the marijuana of the 1969 Woodstock generation;

11. Johnston LD, O'Malley PM, Miech RA, Bachman JG, Schulenberg JE. Monitoring the Future national survey results on drug use, 1975–2015: Overview, key findings on adolescent drug use. Ann Arbor: Institute for Social

Research, The University of Michigan; 2016.
http://www.monitoringthefuture.org/pubs/monographs/
mtf-overview2015.pdf.

12. Rioux, C., Castellanos-Ryan N., Parent, S., Vitaro, F.,
Tremblay, R.E., and Séguin, J.R. Age of Cannabis Use
Onset and Adult Drug Abuse Symptoms: A Prospective
Study of Common Risk Factors and Indirect Effects.
Can J Psychiatry 2018 Jul;63(7):457-464. PubMed
PMID29682999_PubMed Central PMC6099774 Free

13. Galvez-Buccollini, J.A., Proal A.C., Tomaselli V.,
Trachtenberg M., Coconcea C., Chun J., Manschreck
T., Fleming J., Delisi L.E. Association between age at
onset of psychosis and age at onset of cannabis use in
non-affective psychosis. Schizophr Res. 2012 Aug;139(1-
3):157-60. PubMed PMID22727454 PubMed Central
PMC3415971 FREE

14. Hosseini S., and Oremus M. he Effect of Age of Initiation
of Cannabis Use on Psychosis, Depression, and Anxiety
among Youth under 25 Years. Can J Psychiatry. 2019
May;64(5):304-312. PubMED PMID30373388_PubMed
Central PMC6591882 FREE

15. Harvey PD. Smoking Cannabis and Acquired
Impairments in Cognition: Starting Early Seems
Like a Really Bad Idea. Am J Psychiatry. 2019;176(2):90-1.
PubMed PMID: 30704281.

16. Volkow ND, Swanson JM, Evins AE, DeLisi LE, Meier
MH, Gonzalez R, et al. Effects of Cannabis Use on
Human Behavior, Including Cognition, Motivation, and
Psychosis: A Review. JAMA Psychiatry. 2016;73(3):292-7.
PubMed PMID: 26842658. FREE

17. Earleywine M, Luba, R., Slavin, M. N., Farmer, S. & Loflin, M. Don't wake and bake: morning use predicts cannabis problems. . Addict Res Theory. 2016;24:426–30.

18. Heard K, Monte AA, Hoyte CO. Brief Commentary: Consequences of Marijuana-Observations From the Emergency Department. Ann Intern Med. 2019;170(2):124. PubMed PMID: 30615784; PubMed Central PMCID: 6669097. FREE

19. Hall KE, Monte AA, Chang T, Fox J, Brevik C, Vigil DI, et al. Mental Health-related Emergency Department Visits Associated With Cannabis in Colorado. Acad Emerg Med. 2018;25(5):526-37. PubMed PMID: 29476688; PubMed Central PMCID: 5980767. FREE

20. Roberts BA. Legalized Cannabis in Colorado Emergency Departments: A Cautionary Review of Negative Health and Safety Effects. West J Emerg Med. 2019;20(4):557-72. PubMed PMID: 31316694; PubMed Central PMCID: 6625695. FREE

21. Bhattacharyya S, Morrison PD, Fusar-Poli P, Martin-Santos R, Borgwardt S, Winton-Brown T, et al. Opposite effects of delta-9-tetrahydrocannabinol and cannabidiol on human brain function and psychopathology. Neuropsychopharmacology. 2010;35(3):764-74. PubMed PMID: 19924114; PubMed Central PMCID: 3055598. FREE

23. Hjorthoj C, Posselt CM. Delta(9)-tetrahydrocannabinol: harmful even in low doses? Lancet Psychiatry. 2020;7(4):296-7. PubMed PMID: 32197091.

24. Hindley G, Beck K, Borgan F, Ginestet CE, McCutcheon R, Kleinloog D, et al. Psychiatric symptoms caused by cannabis constituents: a systematic review and meta-analysis. Lancet Psychiatry. 2020;7(4):344-53. PubMed PMID: 32197092.

25. Dose-Response Relationship Wikipedia [https://pubmed. ncbi.nlm.nih.gov/32197092/8/21/2020]. Available from: https://en.wikipedia.org/wiki/ Dose–response_relationship.

26. Marconi A, Di Forti M, Lewis CM, Murray RM, Vassos E. Meta-analysis of the Association Between the Level of Cannabis Use and Risk of Psychosis. Schizophr Bull. 2016;42(5):1262-9. PubMed PMID: 26884547; PubMed Central PMCID: 4988731. FREE

27. Ramaekers JG, van Wel JH, Spronk DB, Toennes SW, Kuypers KP, Theunissen EL, et al. Cannabis and tolerance: acute drug impairment as a function of cannabis use history. Sci Rep. 2016;6:26843.PubMed PMID: 27225696; PubMed Central PMCID: 4881034. FREE

28. Curran HV, Brignell C, Fletcher S, Middleton P, Henry J. Cognitive and subjective dose-response effects of acute oral Delta 9-tetrahydrocannabinol (THC) in infrequent cannabis users. Psychopharmacology (Berl). 2002;164(1):61-70. PubMed PMID: 12373420.

29. Ramaekers JG, Kauert G, van Ruitenbeek P, Theunissen EL, Schneider E, Moeller MR. High-potency marijuana impairs executive function and inhibitory motor control. Neuropsychopharmacology. 2006;31(10):2296-303. PubMed PMID: 16572123. FREE

30. Crean RD, Crane NA, Mason BJ. An evidence based review of acute and long-term effects of cannabis use on executive cognitive functions. J Addict Med. 2011;5(1):1-8. PubMed PMID: 21321675; PubMed Central PMCID: 3037578. FREE

31 Bossong MG, van Hell HH, Schubart CD, van Saane W, Iseger TA, Jager G, et al. Acute effects of 9-tetrahydrocannabinol (THC) on resting state brain

function and their modulation by COMT genotype. Eur Neuropsychopharmacol. 2019;29(6):766-76. PubMed PMID: 30975584.

32. Crane NA, Schuster RM, Fusar-Poli P, Gonzalez R. Effects of cannabis on neurocognitive functioning: recent advances, neurodevelopmental influences, and sex differences. Neuropsychol Rev. 2013;23(2):117-37. PubMed PMID: 23129391; PubMed Central PMCID: 3593817. FREE

33. Mortality Risk of COVID-19 Oxford University Access date. 1/11/2021 https://ourworldindata.org/mortality-risk-covid

34. Ortiz-Medina MB, Perea M, Torales J, Ventriglio A, Vitrani G, Aguilar L, et al. Cannabis consumption and psychosis or schizophrenia development. Int J Soc Psychiatry. 2018;64(7):690-704. PubMed PMID: 30442059.

35. Cascini F, Aiello C, Di Tanna G. Increasing delta-9-tetrahydrocannabinol (Delta-9-THC) content in herbal cannabis over time: systematic review and meta-analysis. Curr Drug Abuse Rev. 2012;5(1):32-40. PubMed PMID: 22150622.

36. Smart R, Caulkins JP, Kilmer B, Davenport S, Midgette G. Variation in cannabis potency and prices in a newly legal market: evidence from 30 million cannabis sales in Washington state. Addiction. 2017;112(12):2167-77. PubMed PMID: 28556310; PubMed Central PMCID: 5673542. FREE

37. Wilson J, Freeman TP, Mackie CJ. Effects of increasing cannabis potency on adolescent health. Lancet Child Adolesc Health. 2019;3(2):121-8. PubMed PMID: 30573419.

38. Surgeon General. Available from: https://www.hhs.gov/surgeongeneral/reports-and-publications/addiction-and-substance-misuse/advisory-on-marijuana-use-and-developing-brain/index.html.

39. Stogner JM, Miller BL. Assessing the Dangers of "Dabbing": Mere Marijuana or Harmful New Trend? Pediatrics. 2015;136(1):1-3. PubMed PMID: 26077476.

40. Patrick ME, Miech RA, Kloska DD, Wagner AC, Johnston LD. Trends in Marijuana Vaping and Edible Consumption From 2015 to 2018 Among Adolescents in the US. JAMA Pediatr. 2020. PubMed PMID: 32250422.

41. Schauer GL, Njai R, Grant-Lenzy AM. Modes of marijuana use – smoking, vaping, eating, and dabbing: Results from the 2016 BRFSS in 12 States. Drug Alcohol Depend. 2020;209:107900. PubMed PMID: 32061947.

42. Cannabis concentrates Wikipedia (8-12-20). Available from: https://en.wikipedia.org/wiki/Cannabis_concentrate.

Chapter 4: Marijuana Myths and other important thoughts about Weed: Refs. 43-121
Marijuana is Not Addictive; Marijuana is natural so it can't be bad; Weed is not a gateway drug to harder drugs; There is not enough scientific study of marijuana; Legalization and the public perception of safety; Industry Disinformation; Weed Use Trajectories; Edibles; Poly-Substance Use; Thoughts about Medical Marijuana

43. Koob GF, Volkow ND. Neurobiology of addiction: a neurocircuitry analysis. Lancet Psychiatry. 2016;3(8):760-73. PubMed PMID: 27475769; PubMed Central PMCID: 6135092. FREE

44. Compton WM, Han B, Jones CM, Blanco C. Cannabis use disorders among adults in the United States during a time of increasing use of cannabis. Drug Alcohol Depend. 2019;204:107468. PubMed PMID: 31586809.

45. Yuan M, Kanellopoulos T, Kotbi N. Cannabis use and psychiatric illness in the context of medical marijuana legalization: A clinical perspective. Gen Hosp Psychiatry. 2019;61:82-3. PubMed PMID: 31488324.

46. Hill KP. Marijuana: The Unbiased Truth About The Worlds Most Popular Weed.: Hazelden; 2015. 206 p.

47. Cerda M, Mauro C, Hamilton A, Levy NS, Santaella-Tenorio J, Hasin D, et al. Association Between Recreational Marijuana Legalization in the United States and Changes in Marijuana Use and Cannabis Use Disorder From 2008 to 2016. JAMA Psychiatry. 2019. PubMed PMID: 31722000; PubMed Central PMCID: 6865220. FREE

48. Lope z-Quintero C, Perez de los Cobos J, Hasin DS, Okuda M, Wang S, Grant BF, et al. Probability and predictors of transition from first use to dependence on nicotine, alcohol, cannabis, and cocaine: results of the National Epidemiologic Survey on Alcohol and Related Conditions (NESARC). Drug Alcohol Depend. 2011;115(1-2):120-30. PubMed PMID: 21145178; PubMed Central PMCID: 3069146. FREE

49. Ferland JN, Hurd YL. Deconstructing the neurobiology of cannabis use disorder. Nat Neurosci. 2020. PubMed PMID: 32251385.

50. Chandra S, Radwan MM, Majumdar CG, Church JC, Freeman TP, ElSohly MA. New trends in cannabis potency in USA and Europe during the last decade (2008-2017).

Eur Arch Psychiatry Clin Neurosci. 2019;269(1):5-15. PubMed PMID: 30671616.

51. Bahji A, Stephenson C, Tyo R, Hawken ER, Seitz DP. Prevalence of Cannabis Withdrawal Symptoms Among People With Regular or Dependent Use of Cannabinoids: A Systematic Review and Meta-analysis. JAMA Netw Open. 2020;3(4):e202370. PubMed PMID: 32271390. PubMed Central PMCID: 7146100 FREE

52. American Psychiatric Association. (2013). Diagnostic and statistical manual of mental disorders (5th ed.)

53. Gaston TE, Mendrick DL, Paine MF, Roe AL, Yeung CK. "Natural" is not synonymous with "Safe": Toxicity of Natural Products Alone and in combination with pharmaceutical agents. Regul Toxicol Pharmacol. 2020:104642. PubMed PMID: 32197968.

54. Oleander. Available from: https://en.wikipedia.org/wiki/Nerium.

55. Wolfsbane. Available from: https://en.wikipedia.org/wiki/Aconitum#Toxicology.

56. Craven CB, Wawryk N, Jiang P, Liu Z, Li XF. Pesticides and trace elements in cannabis: Analytical and environmental challenges and opportunities. J Environ Sci (China). 2019;85:82-93. PubMed PMID: 31471034.

57. Atapattu SN, Johnson KRD. Pesticide analysis in cannabis products. J Chromatogr A. 2020;1612:460656. PubMed PMID: 31679712.

58. Maguire WJ, Call CW, Cerbu C, Jambor KL, Benavides-Montes VE. Comprehensive Determination of Unregulated Pesticide Residues in Oregon Cannabis Flower by Liquid Chromatography Paired with Triple Quadrupole Mass Spectrometry and Gas Chromatography

Paired with Triple Quadrupole Mass Spectrometry. J Agric Food Chem. 2019;67(46):12670-4. PubMed PMID: 31398037.

59. Evoy R, Kincl L. Evaluation of Pesticides Found in Oregon Cannabis from 2016 to 2017. Ann Work Expo Health. 2019. PubMed PMID: 31621879.

60. Fergusson DM, Boden JM, Horwood LJ. Cannabis use and other illicit drug use: testing the cannabis gateway hypothesis. Addiction. 2006;101(4):556-69. PubMed PMID: 16548935.

61. Secades-Villa R, Garcia-Rodriguez O, Jin CJ, Wang S, Blanco C. Probability and predictors of the cannabis gateway effect: a national study. Int J Drug Policy. 2015;26(2):135-42. PubMed PMID: 25168081; PubMed Central PMCID: 4291295. FREE

62. Rabiee R, Lundin A, Agardh E, Forsell Y, Allebeck P, Danielsson AK. Cannabis use, subsequent other illicit drug use and drug use disorders: A 16-year follow-up study among Swedish adults. Addict Behav. 2020;106:106390. PubMed PMID: 32179379. FREE

63. Degenhardt L, Hall W, Lynskey M. The relationship between cannabis use and other substance use in the general population. Drug Alcohol Depend. 2001;64(3):319-27. PubMed PMID: 11672946.

64. Kandel D. Stages in adolescent involvement in drug use. Science. 1975;190(4217):912-4. PubMed PMID: 1188374.

65. Cappelli C, Ames SL, Xie B, Pike JR, Stacy AW. Acceptance of Drug Use Mediates Future Hard Drug Use Among At-Risk Adolescent Marijuana, Tobacco, and Alcohol Users. Prev Sci. 2020. PubMed PMID: 32929694.

66. Panlilio LV, Zanettini C, Barnes C, Solinas M, Goldberg SR. Prior exposure to THC increases the addictive effects of nicotine in rats. Neuropsychopharmacology. 2013;38(7):1198-208. PubMed PMID: 23314220; PubMed Central PMCID: 3656362. FREE

67. Lecca D, Scifo A, Pisanu A, Valentini V, Piras G, Sil A, et al. Adolescent cannabis exposure increases heroin reinforcement in rats genetically vulnerable to addiction. Neuropharmacology. 2020;166:107974. PubMed PMID: 32007624.

68. Ishida JH, Zhang AJ, Steigerwald S, Cohen BE, Vali M, Keyhani S. Sources of Information and Beliefs About the Health Effects of Marijuana. J Gen Intern Med. 2020;35(1):153-9. PubMed PMID: 31637640; PubMed Central PMCID: 6957653. FREE

69. Wen H, Hockenberry JM, Druss BG. The Effect of Medical Marijuana Laws on Marijuana-Related Attitude and Perception Among US Adolescents and Young Adults. Prev Sci. 2019;20(2):215-23. PubMed PMID: 29767282.

70. Allen JA, Farrelly MC, Duke JC, Kamyab K, Nonnemaker JM, Wylie S, et al. Perceptions of the relative harmfulness of marijuana and alcohol among adults in Oregon. Prev Med. 2018;109:34-8. PubMed PMID: 29330028.

71. Chadi N, Levy S, Weitzman ER. Moving beyond perceived riskiness: Marijuana-related beliefs and marijuana use in adolescents. Subst Abus. 2019:1-4. PubMed PMID: 31361591.

72. Union of Concerned Scientists- Disinformation Playbook [6-22-20]. Available from: https://www.ucsusa.org/resources/disinformation-playbook.

73. Humphreys K, Hall WD. Reducing the risks of distortion in cannabis research. Addiction. 2020;115(5):799-801. PubMed PMID: 31491039.

74. Windle M, Wiesner M. Trajectories of marijuana use from adolescence to young adulthood: predictors and outcomes. Dev Psychopathol. 2004;16(4):1007-27. PubMed PMID: 15704825.

75. Brook JS, Lee JY, Brown EN, Finch SJ, Brook DW. Developmental trajectories of marijuana use from adolescence to adulthood: personality and social role outcomes. Psychol Rep. 2011;108(2):339-. PubMed PMID: 21675549; PubMed Central PMCID: 3117277. FREE

76. Terry-McElrath YM, O'Malley PM, Johnston LD, Bray BC, Patrick ME, Schulenberg JE. Longitudinal patterns of marijuana use across ages 18-50 in a US national sample: A descriptive examination of predictors and health correlates of repeated measures latent class membership. Drug Alcohol Depend. 2017;171:70-83. PubMed PMID: 28024188; PubMed Central PMCID: 5263048.

77. De Genna NM, Cornelius MD, Goldschmidt L, Day NL. Maternal age and trajectories of cannabis use. Drug Alcohol Depend. 2015;156:199-206. PubMed PMID: 26429727; PubMed Central PMCID: 4633363. FREE

78. Thompson K, Leadbeater B, Ames M, Merrin GJ. Associations Between Marijuana Use Trajectories and Educational and Occupational Success in Young Adulthood. Prev Sci. 2019;20(2):257-69. PubMed PMID: 29704147; PubMed Central PMCID: 6414467. FREE

79. Passarotti AM, Crane NA, Hedeker D, Mermelstein RJ. Longitudinal trajectories of marijuana use from adolescence to young adulthood. Addict Behav.

2015;45:301-8. PubMed PMID: 25792233; PubMed Central PMCID: 4374005. FREE

80. Suerken CK, Reboussin BA, Egan KL, Sutfin EL, Wagoner KG, Spangler J, et al. Marijuana use trajectories and academic outcomes among college students. Drug Alcohol Depend. 2016;162:137-45. PubMed PMID: 27020322; PubMed Central PMCID: 4835174. FREE

81. Arria AM, Caldeira KM, Bugbee BA, Vincent KB, O'Grady KE. The academic consequences of marijuana use during college. Psychol Addict Behav. 2015;29(3):564-75. PubMed PMID: 26237288; PubMed Central PMCID: 4586361. FREE

82. Marmet S, Studer J, Wicki M, Gmel G. Cannabis use disorder trajectories and their prospective predictors in a large population-based sample of young Swiss men. Addiction. 2020. PubMed PMID: 32621560.

83. Hancock-Allen JB, Barker L, VanDyke M, Holmes DB. Notes from the Field: Death Following Ingestion of an Edible Marijuana Product–Colorado, March 2014. MMWR Morb Mortal Wkly Rep. 2015;64(28):771-2. PubMed PMID: 26203632; PubMed Central PMCID: 4584864. FREE

84. Zipursky JS, Bogler OD, Stall NM. Edible cannabis. CMAJ. 2020;192(7):E162. PubMed PMID: 32071107.

85. Zuckermann AME, Williams GC, Battista K, Jiang Y, de Groh M, Leatherdale ST. Prevalence and correlates of youth poly-substance use in the COMPASS study. Addict Behav. 2020;107:106400. PubMed PMID: 32222564.

86. Cairns KE, Yap MB, Pilkington PD, Jorm AF. Risk and protective factors for depression that adolescents can modify: a systematic review and meta-analysis of longitudinal studies. J Affect Disord. 2014;169:61-75. PubMed PMID: 25154536.

87. Kelly AB, Chan GC, Mason WA, Williams JW. The relationship between psychological distress and adolescent polydrug use. Psychol Addict Behav. 2015;29(3):787-93. PubMed PMID: 26415064.

88. Lopez-Quintero C, Granja K, Hawes S, Duperrouzel JC, Pacheco-Colon I, Gonzalez R. Transition to drug co-use among adolescent cannabis users: The role of decision-making and mental health. Addict Behav. 2018;85:43-50. PubMed PMID: 29843040; PubMed Central PMCID: 6740328. FREE

89. Bohnert KM, Walton MA, Resko S, Barry KT, Chermack ST, Zucker RA, et al. Latent class analysis of substance use among adolescents presenting to urban primary care clinics. Am J Drug Alcohol Abuse. 2014;40(1):44-50. PubMed PMID: 24219231; PubMed Central PMCID: 4346305. FREE

90. Maslowsky J, Schulenberg JE, O'Malley PM, Kloska DD. Depressive symptoms, conduct problems, and risk for polysubstance use among adolescents: Results from US national surveys. Ment Health Subst Use. 2013;7(2):157-69. PubMed PMID: 24578719; PubMed Central PMCID: 3932991. FREE

91. Chadi N, Li G, Cerda N, Weitzman ER. Depressive Symptoms and Suicidality in Adolescents Using e-Cigarettes and Marijuana: A Secondary Data Analysis From the Youth Risk Behavior Survey. J Addict Med. 2019;13(5):362-5. PubMed PMID: 30688723.

92. Werner AK, Koumans EH, Chatham-Stephens K, Salvatore PP, Armatas C, Byers P, et al. Hospitalizations and Deaths Associated with EVALI. N Engl J Med. 2020;382(17):1589-98. PubMed PMID: 32320569.

93. Vaping EVALI CDC [4-24-20]. Available from: https://www.cdc.gov/tobacco/basic_information/e-cigarettes/severe-lung-disease.html.

94. Kowitt SD, Osman A, Meernik C, Zarkin GA, Ranney LM, Martin J, et al. Vaping cannabis among adolescents: prevalence and associations with tobacco use from a cross-sectional study in the USA. BMJ Open. 2019;9(6):e028535. PubMed PMID: 31196904; PubMed Central PMCID: 6585821. FREE

95. Noorbakhsh S, Afzali MH, Boers E, Conrod PJ. Cognitive Function Impairments Linked to Alcohol and Cannabis Use During Adolescence: A Study of Gender Differences. Front Hum Neurosci. 2020;14:95. PubMed PMID: 32317950; PubMed Central PMCID: 7154290. FREE

96. Wade NE, Thomas AM, Gruber SA, Tapert SF, Filbey FM, Lisdahl KM. Binge and Cannabis Co-Use Episodes in Relation to White Matter Integrity in Emerging Adults. Cannabis Cannabinoid Res. 2020;5(1):62-72. PubMed PMID: 32322677; PubMed Central PMCID: 7173670. FREE

97. Ramaekers JG. Driving Under the Influence of Cannabis: An Increasing Public Health Concern. JAMA. 2018;319(14):1433-4. PubMed PMID: 29582068.

98. Sayer G, Ialomiteanu A, Stoduto G, Wickens CM, Mann RE, Le Foll B, et al. Increased collision risk among drivers who report driving after using alcohol and after using cannabis. Can J Public Health. 2014;105(1):e92-3. PubMed PMID: 24735704; PubMed Central PMCID: 6972259. FREE

99. Whiting PF, Wolff RF, Deshpande S, Di Nisio M, Duffy S, Hernandez AV, et al. Cannabinoids for Medical Use: A Systematic Review and Meta-analysis. JAMA. 2015;313(24):2456-73. PubMed PMID: 26103030.

100. Kesner AJ, Lovinger DM. Cannabinoids, Endocannabinoids and Sleep. Front Mol Neurosci. 2020;13:125. PubMed PMID: 32774241; PubMed Central PMCID: 7388834. FREE

101. Wilsey B, Marcotte T, Deutsch R, Gouaux B, Sakai S, Donaghe H. Low-dose vaporized cannabis significantly improves neuropathic pain. J Pain. 2013;14(2):136-48. PubMed PMID: 23237736; PubMed Central PMCID: 3566631. FREE

102. Raymundi AM, da Silva TR, Sohn JMB, Bertoglio LJ, Stern CA. Effects of (9)-tetrahydrocannabinol on aversive memories and anxiety: a review from human studies. BMC Psychiatry. 2020;20(1):420. PubMed PMID: 32842985.

103. Andreae MH, Carter GM, Shaparin N, Suslov K, Ellis RJ, Ware MA, et al. Inhaled Cannabis for Chronic Neuropathic Pain: A Meta-analysis of Individual Patient Data. J Pain. 2015;16(12):1221-32. PubMed PMID: 26362106; PubMed Central PMCID: 4666747. FREE

104. Nielsen S, Germanos R, Weier M, Pollard J, Degenhardt L, Hall W, et al. The Use of Cannabis and Cannabinoids in Treating Symptoms of Multiple Sclerosis: a Systematic Review of Reviews. Curr Neurol Neurosci Rep. 2018;18(2):8. PubMed PMID: 29442178.

105. Szejko N, Fremer C, Muller-Vahl KR. Cannabis Improves Obsessive-Compulsive Disorder-Case Report and Review of the Literature. Front Psychiatry. 2020;11:681. PubMed PMID: 32848902; PubMed Central PMCID: 7396551. FREE

106. Billnitzer A, Jankovic J. Current Management of Tics and Tourette Syndrome: Behavioral, Pharmacologic, and

Surgical Treatments. Neurotherapeutics. 2020. PubMed PMID: 32856174.

107. Dibba P, Li AA, Cholankeril G, Ali Khan M, Kim D, Ahmed A. Potential Mechanisms Influencing the Inverse Relationship Between Cannabis and Nonalcoholic Fatty Liver Disease: A Commentary. Nutr Metab Insights. 2019;12 PubMed PMID: 31308686; PubMed Central PMCID: 6612909. FREE

108. Adejumo AC, Alliu S, Ajayi TO, Adejumo KL, Adegbala OM, Onyeakusi NE, et al. Cannabis use is associated with reduced prevalence of non-alcoholic fatty liver disease: A cross-sectional study. PLoS One. 2017;12(4):e0176416. PubMed PMID: 28441459; PubMed Central PMCID: 5404771. FREE

109. Adejumo AC, Adegbala OM, Adejumo KL, Bukong TN. Reduced Incidence and Better Liver Disease Outcomes among Chronic HCV Infected Patients Who Consume Cannabis. Can J Gastroenterol Hepatol. 2018;2018:9430953. PubMed PMID: 30345261; PubMed Central PMCID: 6174743. FREE

110. Cuttler C, Spradlin A, Cleveland MJ, Craft RM. Short- and Long-Term Effects of Cannabis on Headache and Migraine. J Pain. 2019. PubMed PMID: 31715263.

111. Erridge S, Miller M, Gall T, Costanzo A, Pacchetti B, Sodergren MH. A Comprehensive Patient and Public Involvement Program Evaluating Perception of Cannabis-Derived Medicinal Products in the Treatment of Acute Postoperative Pain, Nausea, and Vomiting Using a Qualitative Thematic Framework. Cannabis Cannabinoid Res. 2020;5(1):73-80. PubMed PMID: 32322678; PubMed Central PMCID: 7173671. FREE

112. Adhiyaman V, Arshad S. Cannabis for intractable nausea after bilateral cerebellar stroke. J Am Geriatr Soc. 2014;62(6):1199. PubMed PMID: 24925562.

113. Smith LA, Azariah F, Lavender VT, Stoner NS, Bettiol S. Cannabinoids for nausea and vomiting in adults with cancer reeiving chemotherapy. Cochrane Database Syst Rev. 2015;(11):CD009464. PubMed PMID: 26561338; PubMed Central PMCID: 6931414. FREE

114. Shar key KA, Darmani NA, Parker LA. Regulation of nausea and vomiting by cannabinoids and the endocannabinoid system. Eur J Pharmacol. 2014;722:134-46. PubMed PMID: 24184696; PubMed Central PMCID: 3883513. FREE

115. Black N, Stockings E, Campbell G, Tran LT, Zagic D, Hall WD, et al. Cannabinoids for the treatment of mental disorders and symptoms of mental disorders: a systematic review and meta-analysis. Lancet Psychiatry. 2019;6(12):995-1010. PubMedPMID: 31672337; PubMed Central PMCID: 6949116. FREE

116. Nugent SM, Morasco BJ, O'Neil ME, Freeman M, Low A, Kondo K, et al. The Effects of Cannabis Among Adults With Chronic Pain and an Overview of General Harms: A Systematic Review. Ann Intern Med. 2017;167(5):319-31. Epub 2017/08/15. doi: 10.7326/M17-0155. PubMed PMID: 28806817. FREE

117. Pratt M., Stevens A.,Thuku M., Butler C., Skidmore B., Wieland L.S., Clemons M., Kanji M., Hutton B. Benefits and harms of medical cannabis: a scoping review of systematic reviews. Syst Rev. 2019 Dec 10;8(1):320. PubMed PMID31823819_PubMed Central PMC6905063 FREE

118. Dronabinol Wikipedia [8/29/2020]. Available from: https://en.wikipedia.org/wiki/Dronabinol.

119. Savitex Wikipedia [9/10/2020]. Available from: https://en.wikipedia.org/wiki/Nabiximols.

120. Nabilone-Wikipedia [8/29/2020]. Available from: https://en.wikipedia.org/wiki/Nabilone.

121. Epidiolex Epidiolex.com [9/12/2020]. Available from: https://www.epidiolex.com/.

Chapter 5: Biological, Biochemical, and Genetic Basics: Refs. 122-228

Tetrahydrocannabinol, THC and Cannabidiol, CBD; Tolerance to THC; Common Genetics and Weed; DNA: The Long Stringy Stuff; Four Important Genes; Epigenetics; Cytochrome P450s: Cannabis, Prescription Drug interactions and Metabolism.

122. THC Wikipedia. Available from: https://en.wikipedia.org/wiki/Tetrahydrocannabinol.

123. Hanus LO, Meyer SM, Munoz E, Taglialatela-Scafati O, Appendino G. Phytocannabinoids: a unified critical inventory. Nat Prod Rep. 2016;33(12):1357-92. PubMed PMID: 27722705

124. Sideli L, Trotta G, Spinazzola E, La Cascia C, Di Forti M. Adverse effects of heavy cannabis use: even plants can harm the brain. Pain. 2020. PubMed PMID: 32804835.

125. CBD Wikipedia. Available from: https://en.wikipedia.org/wiki/Cannabidiol

126. Batalla A, Janssen H, Gangadin SS, Bossong MG. The Potential of Cannabidiol as a Treatment for Psychosis and Addiction: Who Benefits Most? A Systematic Review.

J Clin Med. 2019;8(7). PubMed PMID: 31330972; PubMed Central PMCID: 6678854. FREE

127. Zeyl V, Sawyer K, Wightman RS. What Do You Know About Maryjane? A Systematic Review of the Current Data on the THC:CBD Ratio. Subst Use Misuse. 2020:1-5. PubMed PMID: 32124675. FREE

128. Cannabigerol Wikipedia [8/21-2020]. Available from: https://en.wikipedia.org/wiki/Cannabigerol.

129. Cannabis sativa Wikipedia [8/8/2020]. Available from: https://en.wikipedia.org/wiki/Cannabis_sativa.

130. Cannabis indica Wikipedia [8/8/2020]. Available from: https://en.wikipedia.org/wiki/Cannabis_indica.

131. Morland J, Bramness JG. Delta9-tetrahydrocannabinol (THC) is present in the body between smoking sessions in occasional non-daily cannabis users. Forensic Sci Int. 2020;309:110188. PubMed PMID: 32120192.

132. Howlett AC, Abood ME. CB1 and CB2 Receptor Pharmacology. Adv Pharmacol. 2017;80:169-206. PubMed PMID: 28826534; PubMed Central PMCID: 5812699. FREE

133. CNR1 CB1 Entrez gene. Available from: https://www.ncbi.nlm.nih.gov/gene/1268.

134. CNR2 CB2 Entrez gene. Available from: https://www.ncbi.nlm.nih.gov/gene/1269

135. CNR1 Cannabinoid receptor IUPHAR/BPS Guide to Pharmacology [4/6/2020]. Available from: https://www.guidetopharmacology.org/

136. Pava MJ, Makriyannis A, Lovinger DM. Endocannabinoid Signaling Regulates Sleep Stability.

PLoS One. 2016;11(3):e0152473. PubMed PMID: 27031992; PubMed Central PMCID: 4816426. FREE

137. Dopamine Wikipedia. Available from: https://en.wikipedia.org/wiki/Dopamine.

138. Oleson EB, Cheer JF. A brain on cannabinoids: the role of dopamine release in reward seeking. Cold Spring Harb Perspect Med. 2012;2(8). PubMed PMID: 22908200; PubMed Central PMCID: 3405830. FREE

139. Anandamide Wikipedia. Available from: https://en.wikipedia.org/wiki/Anandamide.

140. Volkow ND, Wang GJ, Telang F, Fowler JS, Alexoff D, Logan J, et al. Decreased dopamine brain reactivity in marijuana abusers is associated with negative emotionality and addiction severity. Proc Natl Acad Sci U S A. 2014;111(30):E3149-56. PubMed PMID: 25024177; PubMed Central PMCID: 4121778. FREE

141. van de Giessen E, Weinstein JJ, Cassidy CM, Haney M, Dong Z, Ghazzaoui R, et al. Deficits in striatal dopamine release in cannabis dependence. Mol Psychiatry. 2017;22(1):68-75. PubMed PMID: 27001613; PubMed Central PMCID: 5033654. FREE

142. Bloomfield MA, Ashok AH, Volkow ND, Howes OD. The effects of Delta(9)-tetrahydrocannabinol on the dopamine system. Nature. 2016;539(7629):369-77. PubMed PMID: 27853201; PubMed Central PMCID: 5123717. FREE

143. Ramaekers JG, Mason NL, Theunissen EL. Blunted highs: Pharmacodynamic and behavioral models of cannabis tolerance. Eur Neuropsychopharmacol. 2020;36:191-205. PubMed PMID: 32014378.

144. Hall W, Degenhardt L. Adverse health effects of non-medical cannabis use. Lancet. 2009;374(9698):1383-91. PubMed PMID: 19837255.

145. Executive Functions Wikipedia. Available from: https://en.wikipedia.org/wiki/Executive_functions.

146. Alcaro A, Huber R, Panksepp J. Behavioral functions of the mesolimbic dopaminergic system: an affective neuroethological perspective. Brain Res Rev. 2007;56(2):283-321. PubMed PMID: 17905440; PubMed Central PMCID: 2238694. FREE

147. Volkow ND, Gillespie H, Mullani N, Tancredi L, Grant C, Valentine A, et al. Brain glucose metabolism in chronic marijuana users at baseline and during marijuana intoxication. Psychiatry Res. 1996;67(1):29-38. PubMed PMID: 8797240.

148. Peters KZ, Oleson EB, Cheer JF. A Brain on Cannabinoids: The Role of Dopamine Release in Reward Seeking and Addiction. Cold Spring Harb Perspect Med. 2020. PubMed PMID: 31964646.

149. Polli L, Schwan R, Albuisson E, Malbos L, Angioi-Duprez K, Laprevote V, et al. Oscillatory potentials abnormalities in regular cannabis users: Amacrine cells dysfunction as a marker of central dopaminergic modulation. Prog Neuropsychopharmacol Biol Psychiatry. 2020:110083. PubMed PMID: 32860840.

150. Chetia S, Borah G. Delta 9-Tetrahydrocannabinol Toxicity and Validation of Cannabidiol on Brain Dopamine Levels: An Assessment on Cannabis Duplicity. Nat Prod Bioprospect. 2020. PubMed PMID: 32860199.

151. Mesolimbic pathway -Wikipedia [8/31/2020]. Available from: https://en.wikipedia.org/wiki/Mesolimbic_pathway.

152. Bloomfield MA, Morgan CJ, Kapur S, Curran HV, Howes OD. The link between dopamine function and apathy in cannabis users: an [18F]-DOPA PET imaging study. Psychopharmacology (Berl). 2014;231(11):2251-9. PubMed PMID: 24696078.

153. Abood ME, Martin BR. Neurobiology of marijuana abuse. Trends Pharmacol Sci. 1992;13(5):201-6. PubMed PMID: 1604713.

154. Compton DR, Dewey WL, Martin BR. Cannabis dependence and tolerance production. Adv Alcohol Subst Abuse. 1990;9(1-2):129-47. PubMed PMID: 2165734.

155. Nowlan R, Cohen S. Tolerance to marijuana: heart rate and subjective "high". Clin Pharmacol Ther. 1977;22(5 Pt 1):550-6. PubMed PMID: 913022.

156. Gregor Mendel Wikipedia [9/26/2020]. Available from: https://en.wikipedia.org/wiki/Gregor_Mendel.

157. Becker KG. The common variants/multiple disease hypothesis of common complex genetic disorders. Med Hypotheses. 2004;62(2):309-17. PubMed PMID: 14962646.

158. SNPedia Cannabis SNPS. Available from: https://www.snpedia.com/index.php/Cannabis.

159. Gutleb DR, Roos C, Noll A, Ostner J, Schulke O. COMT Val(158) Met moderates the link between rank and aggression in a non-human primate. Genes Brain Behav. 2018;17(4):e12443. PubMed PMID: 29194954.

160. Quinn PD, Harden KP. Differential changes in impulsivity and sensation seeking and the escalation

of substance use from adolescence to early adulthood. Dev Psychopathol. 2013;25(1):223-39. PubMed PMID: 22824055; PubMed Central PMCID: 3967723. FREE

161. Ehlers CL, Slutske WS, Lind PA, Wilhelmsen KC. Association between single nucleotide polymorphisms in the cannabinoid receptor gene (CNR1) and impulsivity in southwest California Indians. Twin Res Hum Genet. 2007;10(6):805-11. PubMed PMID: 18179391.

162. Colonna V, Pagani L, Xue Y, Tyler-Smith C. A world in a grain of sand: human history from genetic data. Genome Biol. 2011;12(11):234. PubMed PMID: 22104725; PubMed Central PMCID: 3334592. FREE

163. Jang SK, Saunders G, Liu M, andMe Research T, Jiang Y, Liu DJ, et al. Genetic correlation, pleiotropy, and causal associations between substance use and psychiatric disorder. Psychol Med. 2020:1-11. PubMed PMID: 32762793.

164. CNR1 3D SWISS MODEL [4-26-20]. Available from: https://swissmodel.expasy.org/repository/md5/0c17ebaa15fc6b73f10275d6230f55f0.

165. Hopfer CJ, Young SE, Purcell S, Crowley TJ, Stallings MC, Corley RP, et al. Cannabis receptor haplotype associated with fewer cannabis dependence symptoms in adolescents. Am J Med Genet B Neuropsychiatr Genet. 2006;141B(8):895-901. PubMed PMID: 16917946; PubMed Central PMCID: 2564870. FREE

166. CNR1 rs806368 SNPedia [4/6/20]. Available from: https://www.snpedia.com/index.php/Rs806368.

167. Agrawal A, Wetherill L, Dick DM, Xuei X, Hinrichs A, Hesselbrock V, et al. Evidence for association between

polymorphisms in the cannabinoid receptor 1
(CNR1) gene and cannabis dependence. Am J Med
Genet B Neuropsychiatr Genet. 2009;150B(5):736-40.
PubMed PMID: 19016476; PubMed Central PMCID:
2703788. FREE

168. Hill SY, Jones BL, Steinhauer SR, Zezza N, Stiffler
S. Longitudinal predictors of cannabis use and
dependence in offspring from families at ultra high risk
for alcohol dependence and in control families. Am J
Med Genet B Neuropsychiatr Genet. 2016;171B(3):383-
95. PubMed PMID: 26756393; PubMed Central PMCID:
5444658. FREE

169. Schacht JP, Hutchison KE, Filbey FM. Associations
between cannabinoid receptor-1 (CNR1) variation and
hippocampus and amygdala volumes in heavy cannabis
users. Neuropsychopharmacology. 2012;37(11):2368-
76. PubMed PMID: 22669173; PubMed Central PMCID:
3442352. FREE

170. Marcos M, Pastor I, de la Calle C, Barrio-Real L, Laso FJ,
Gonzalez-Sarmiento R. Cannabinoid receptor 1 gene is
associated with alcohol dependence. Alcohol Clin Exp
Res. 2012;36(2):267-71. PubMed PMID: 22085192.

171. Chen X, Williamson VS, An SS, Hettema JM, Aggen
SH, Neale MC, et al. Cannabinoid receptor 1 gene
association with nicotine dependence. Arch Gen
Psychiatry. 2008;65(7):816-24. PubMed PMID: 18606954;
PubMed Central PMCID: 2733353. FREE

172. Zuo L, Kranzler HR, Luo X, Yang BZ, Weiss R, Brady
K, et al. Interaction between two independent CNR1
variants increases risk for cocaine dependence in
European Americans: a replication study in family-
based sample and population-based sample.

Neuropsychopharmacology. 2009;34(6):1504-13. PubMed PMID: 19052543; PubMed Central PMCID: 2879626. FREE

173. Clarke TK, Bloch PJ, Ambrose-Lanci LM, Ferraro TN, Berrettini WH, Kampman KM, et al. Further evidence for association of polymorphisms in the CNR1 gene with cocaine addiction: confirmation in an independent sample and meta-analysis. Addict Biol. 2013;18(4):702-8. PubMed PMID: 21790903; PubMed Central PMCID: 3223560. FREE

174. Jaeger JP, Mattevi VS, Callegari-Jacques SM, Hutz MH. Cannabinoid type-1 receptor gene polymorphisms are associated with central obesity in a Southern Brazilian population. Dis Markers. 2008;25(1):67-74. PubMed PMID: 18776593; PubMed Central PMCID: 3827795. FREE

175. Palmer, R.H.C, McGeary, J.E., Knopik, V.S., Bidwell, L.C., Metrik, J.M CNR1 and FAAH variation and affective states induced by marijuana smoking. Am J Drug Alcohol Abuse. 2019;45(5):514-526. PubMed PMID31184938 PubMed Central PMC6931041 FREE

176. Lu AT, Ogdie MN, Jarvelin MR, Moilanen IK, Loo SK, McCracken JT, et al. Association of the cannabinoid receptor gene (CNR1) with ADHD and post-traumatic stress disorder. Am J Med Genet B Neuropsychiatr Genet. 2008;147B(8):1488-94. PubMed PMID: 18213623; PubMed Central PMCID: 2685476. FREE

177. Herman AI, Kranzler HR, Cubells JF, Gelernter J, Covault J. Association study of the CNR1 gene exon 3 alternative promoter region polymorphisms and substance dependence. Am J Med Genet B Neuropsychiatr Genet.

2006;141B(5):499-503. PubMed PMID: 16741937; PubMed Central PMCID: 2574012. FREE

178. COMT 3D SWISS MODEL [4-26-20]. Available from: https://swissmodel.expasy.org/repository/md5/ e92814c4c1d9a88463dc4ef61a0d0988.

179. Radhakrishnan R, Wilkinson ST, D'Souza DC. Gone to Pot – A Review of the Association between Cannabis and Psychosis. Front Psychiatry. 2014;5:54. PubMed PMID: 24904437; PubMed Central PMCID: 4033190. FREE

180. Tartar JL, Cabrera D, Knafo S, Thomas JD, Antonio J, Peacock CA. The "Warrior" COMT Val/Met Genotype Occurs in Greater Frequencies in Mixed Martial Arts Fighters Relative to Controls. J Sports Sci Med. 2020;19(1):38-42. PubMed PMID: 32132825; PubMed Central PMCID: 7039020. FREE

181. Caspi A, Moffitt TE, Cannon M, McClay J, Murray R, Harrington H, et al. Moderation of the effect of adolescent-onset cannabis use on adult psychosis by a functional polymorphism in the catechol-O-methyltransferase gene: longitudinal evidence of a gene X environment interaction. Biol Psychiatry. 2005;57(10):1117-27. PubMed PMID: 15866551.

182. Bosia M, Buonocore M, Bechi M, Stere LM, Silvestri MP, Inguscio E, et al. Schizophrenia, cannabis use and Catechol-O-Methyltransferase (COMT): Modeling the interplay on cognition. Prog Neuropsychopharmacol Biol Psychiatry. 2019;92:363-8. PubMed PMID: 30790675.

183. Lodhi RJ, Wang Y, Rossolatos D, MacIntyre G, Bowker A, Crocker C, et al. Investigation of the COMT Val158Met variant association with age of onset of psychosis, adjusting for cannabis use. Brain Behav.

2017;7(11):e00850. PubMed PMID: 29201551; PubMed Central PMCID: 5698868. FREE

184. Pearson NT, Berry JH. Cannabis and Psychosis Through the Lens of DSM-5. Int J Environ Res Public Health. 2019;16(21). PubMed PMID: 31661851; PubMed Central PMCID: 6861931. FREE

185. Cosker E, Schwitzer T, Ramoz N, Ligier F, Lalanne L, Gorwood P, et al. The effect of interactions between genetics and cannabis use on neurocognition. A review. Prog Neuropsychopharmacol Biol Psychiatry. 2018;82:95-106. PubMed PMID: 29191570.

186. COMT rs4680 SNPedia [4-11-20]. Available from: https://www.snpedia.com/index.php/Rs4680.

187. DRD2 Entrez Gene [2-26-20]. Available from: https://www.ncbi.nlm.nih.gov/gene/1813.

188. DRD2 3D structure SWISS MODEL [4-26-20]. Available from: https://swissmodel.expasy.org/repository/md5/18e89a4dd87388f86806f1dee3865a4d.

189. Bhatia A, Saadabadi A. Biochemistry, Dopamine Receptors. StatPearls. Treasure Island (FL)2020.

190. Dopamine receptors Wikipedia [4-26-20]. Available from: https://en.wikipedia.org/wiki/Dopamine_receptor.

191. Lopez-Morales P, Flores-Funes D, Sanchez-Migallon EG, Liron-Ruiz RJ, Aguayo-Albasini JL. Genetic Factors Associated with Postoperative Nausea and Vomiting: a Systematic Review. J Gastrointest Surg. 2018;22(9):1645-51. PubMed PMID: 29725907.

192. Agrawal A, Lynskey MT. Candidate genes for cannabis use disorders: findings, challenges and directions. Addiction. 2009;104(4):518-32.

PubMed PMID: 19335651; PubMed Central PMCID: 2703791. FREE

193. Colizzi M, Iyegbe C, Powell J, Ursini G, Porcelli A, Bonvino A, et al. Interaction Between Functional Genetic Variation of DRD2 and Cannabis Use on Risk of Psychosis. Schizophr Bull. 2015;41(5):1171-82. PubMed PMID: 25829376; PubMed Central PMCID: 4535639. FREE

194. Sasabe T, Furukawa A, Matsusita S, Higuchi S, Ishiura S. Association analysis of the dopamine receptor D2 (DRD2) SNP rs1076560 in alcoholic patients. Neurosci Lett. 2007;412(2):139-42. PubMed PMID: 17196743.

195. DRD2 SNP Rs1076560 SNPedia [4-26-20]. Available from: https://www.snpedia.com/index.php/Rs1076560.

196. Klaus K, Butler K, Curtis F, Bridle C, Pennington K. The effect of ANKK1 Taq1A and DRD2 C957T polymorphisms on executive function: A systematic review and meta-analysis. Neurosci Biobehav Rev. 2019;100:224-36. PubMed PMID: 30836122.

197. Klaus K, Butler K, Durrant SJ, Ali M, Inglehearn CF, Hodgson TL, et al. The effect of COMT Val158Met and DRD2 C957T polymorphisms on executive function and the impact of early life stress. Brain Behav. 2017;7(5):e00695. PubMed PMID: 28523234; PubMed Central PMCID: 5434197. FREE

198. Rodriguez-Jimenez R, Hoenicka J, Jimenez-Arriero MA, Ponce G, Bagney A, Aragues M, et al. Performance in the Wisconsin Card Sorting Test and the C957T polymorphism of the DRD2 gene in healthy volunteers. Neuropsychobiology. 2006;54(3):166-70. PubMed PMID: 17230034.

199. Liu L, Fan D, Ding N, Hu Y, Cai G, Wang L, et al. The relationship between DRD2 gene polymorphisms (C957T and C939T) and schizophrenia: a meta-analysis. Neurosci Lett. 2014;583:43-8. PubMed PMID: 25240594.

200. Jutras-Aswad D, Jacobs MM, Yiannoulos G, Roussos P, Bitsios P, Nomura Y, et al. Cannabis-dependence risk relates to synergism between neuroticism and proenkephalin SNPs associated with amygdala gene expression: case-control study. PLoS One. 2012;7(6):e39243. PubMed PMID: 22745721; PubMed Central PMCID: 3382183. FREE

201. DRD2 rs6277 SNPedia [4-26-20]. Available from: https://www.snpedia.com/index.php/Rs6277.

202. FAAH Wikipedia https://en.wikipedia.org/wiki/Fatty_acid_amide_hydrolase

203. Ahn K, Johnson DS, Cravatt BF. Fatty acid amide hydrolase as a potential therapeutic target for the treatment of pain and CNS disorders. Expert Opin Drug Discov. 2009;4(7):763-84. PubMed PMID: 20544003; PubMed Central PMCID: 2882713. FREE

204. Habib AM, Okorokov AL, Hill MN, Bras JT, Lee MC, Li S, et al. Microdeletion in a FAAH pseudogene identified in a patient with high anandamide concentrations and pain insensitivity. Br J Anaesth. 2019;123(2):e249-e53. PubMed PMID: 30929760; PubMed Central PMCID: 6676009. FREE

205. Sipe J.C., Chiang K., Gerber A.L., Beutler E., and Cravatt B.F. A missense mutation in human fatty acid amide hydrolase associated with problem drug use. Proc Natl Acad Sci U S A. 2002 Jun 11;99(12):8394-9. PubMed PMID12060782 PubMed Central PMC123078 FREE

206. Melroy-Greif WE, Wilhelmsen KC, Ehlers CL. Genetic variation in FAAH is associated with cannabis use disorders in a young adult sample of Mexican Americans. Drug Alcohol Depend. 2016;166:249-53. PubMed PMID: 27394933; PubMed Central PMCID: 4983484. FREE

207. Jacobson MR, Watts JJ, Da Silva T, Tyndale RF, Rusjan PM, Houle S, et al. Fatty acid amide hydrolase is lower in young cannabis users. Addict Biol. 2020:e12872. PubMed PMID: 31960544.

208. D'Souza DC, Cortes-Briones J, Creatura G, Bluez G, Thurnauer H, Deaso E, et al. Efficacy and safety of a fatty acid amide hydrolase inhibitor (PF-04457845) in the treatment of cannabis withdrawal and dependence in men: a double-blind, placebo-controlled, parallel group, phase 2a single-site randomised controlled trial. Lancet Psychiatry. 2019;6(1):35-45. PubMed PMID: 30528676.

209. Haughey HM, Marshall E, Schacht JP, Louis A, Hutchison KE. Marijuana withdrawal and craving: influence of the cannabinoid receptor 1 (CNR1) and fatty acid amide hydrolase (FAAH) genes. Addiction. 2008;103(10):1678-86. PubMed PMID: 18705688; PubMed Central PMCID: 2873690. FREE

210. Filbey FM, Schacht JP, Myers US, Chavez RS, Hutchison KE. Individual and additive effects of the CNR1 and FAAH genes on brain response to marijuana cues. Neuropsychopharmacology. 2010;35(4):967-75. PubMed PMID: 20010552; PubMed Central PMCID: 2820137. FREE

211. Schacht JP, Selling RE, Hutchison KE. Intermediate cannabis dependence phenotypes and the FAAH C385A

variant: an exploratory analysis. Psychopharmacology
(Berl). 2009;203(3):511-7. PubMed PMID: 19002671;
PubMed Central PMCID: 2863054. FREE

212. Campos AC, Moreira FA, Gomes FV, Del Bel EA,
Guimaraes FS. Multiple mechanisms involved in the
large-spectrum therapeutic potential of cannabidiol
in psychiatric disorders. Philos Trans R Soc Lond B
Biol Sci. 2012;367(1607):3364-78. Epub 2012/10/31.
doi: 10.1098/rstb.2011.0389. PubMed PMID: 23108553;
PubMed Central PMCID: 3481531. FREE

213. Gunduz-Cinar O, Hill MN, McEwen BS,
Holmes A. Amygdala FAAH and anandamide: mediating
protection and recovery from stress. Trends Pharmacol
Sci. 2013;34(11):637-44. Epub 2013/12/12. doi: 10.1016/j.
tips.2013.08.008. PubMed PMID: 24325918; PubMed
Central PMCID: 4169112. FREE

214. FAAH rs324420 SNPedia [4-11-20]. Available from:
https://www.snpedia.com/index.php/Rs324420.

215. Hindocha C, Quattrone D, Freeman TP, Murray RM,
Mondelli V, Breen G, et al. Do AKT1, COMT and FAAH
influence reports of acute cannabis intoxication
experiences in patients with first episode psychosis,
controls and young adult cannabis users? Transl
Psychiatry. 2020;10(1):143. PubMed PMID: 32398646.

216. Di Forti M, Iyegbe C, Sallis H, Kolliakou A, Falcone
MA, Paparelli A, et al. Confirmation that the AKT1
(rs2494732) genotype influences the risk of psychosis
in cannabis users. Biol Psychiatry. 2012;72(10):811-6.
PubMed PMID: 22831980.

217. Szutorisz H, Hurd YL. High times for cannabis:
Epigenetic imprint and its legacy on brain and behavior.

Neurosci Biobehav Rev. 2018;85:93-101. PubMed PMID: 28506926; PubMed Central PMCID: 5682234. FREE

218. Osborne AJ, Pearson JF, Noble AJ, Gemmell NJ, Horwood LJ, Boden JM, et al. Genome-wide DNA methylation analysis of heavy cannabis exposure in a New Zealand longitudinal cohort. Transl Psychiatry. 2020;10(1):114. PubMed PMID: 32321915; PubMed Central PMCID: 7176736. FREE

219. Epigenetics Wikkipedia Access date 1-11-2021 https:// en.wikipedia.org/wiki/Epigenetics

220. Prini P, Rusconi F, Zamberletti E, Gabaglio M, Penna F, Fasano M, et al. Adolescent THC exposure in female rats leads to cognitive deficits through a mechanism involving chromatin modifications in the prefrontal cortex. J Psychiatry Neurosci. 2017;42(6):170082. PubMed PMID: 29022873.

221. Wanner, N.M., Colwell, M.L., and Faulk C. The epigenetic legacy of illicit drugs: developmental exposures and late-life phenotypes. Environ Epigenet. 2019 Nov 13;5(4) PubMed PMID31777665 PubMed Central PMC6875650 FREE

222. Smith, A., Kaufman, F., Sandy, M.S., Cardenas, A. Cannabis Exposure During Critical Windows of Development: Epigenetic and Molecular Pathways Implicated in Neuropsychiatric Disease. Curr Environ Health Rep. 2020 Sep;7(3):325-342. PubMed PMID32441004 PubMed Central PMC7458902 FREE

223. Cytochrome P450 Wikipedia [9/14/2020]. Available from: https://en.wikipedia.org/wiki/Cytochrome_P450.

224. Stout SM, Cimino NM. Exogenous cannabinoids as substrates, inhibitors, and inducers of human drug

metabolizing enzymes: a systematic review. Drug Metab Rev. 2014;46(1):86-95. PubMed PMID: 24160757.

225. Watanabe K, Yamaori S, Funahashi T, Kimura T, Yamamoto I. Cytochrome P450 enzymes involved in the metabolism of tetrahydrocannabinols and cannabinol by human hepatic microsomes. Life Sci. 2007;80(15):1415-9. PubMed PMID: 17303175.

226. Medical Cannabis Adverse Effects & Drug Interactions District of Columbia Dept of Health [9/14/2020]. Available from: District of Columbia Dept of Health

227. Damkier P, Lassen D, Christensen MMH, Madsen KG, Hellfritzsch M, Pottegard A. Interaction between warfarin and cannabis. Basic Clin Pharmacol Toxicol. 2019;124(1):28-31. PubMed PMID: 30326170.

228. Cox EJ, Maharao N, Patilea-Vrana G, Unadkat JD, Rettie AE, McCune JS, et al. A marijuana-drug interaction primer: Precipitants, pharmacology, and pharmacokinetics. Pharmacol Ther. 2019;201:25-38. PubMed PMID: 31071346; PubMed Central PMCID: 6708768. FREE

Chapter 6: Brain Stuff: Refs. 229-349
Brain Development and Marijuana; Brain Imaging, Cognition, Memory, and IQ

229. The Brain Wikipedia [5-6-20]. Available from: https://en.wikipedia.org/wiki/Human_brain.

230. Cetacean intelligence Wikipedia [5-6-20]. https://en.wikipedia.org/wiki/Cetacean_intelligence

231. Gogtay N, Giedd JN, Lusk L, Hayashi KM, Greenstein D, Vaituzis AC, et al. Dynamic mapping of human cortical development during childhood through early adulthood.

Proc Natl Acad Sci U S A. 2004;101(21):8174-9. PubMed PMID: 15148381; PubMed Central PMCID: 419576. FREE

232. Brain Development Wikipedia [5-6-20]. Available from: https://en.wikipedia.org/wiki/Human_brain_development_timeline.

233. Johnson SB, Blum RW, Giedd JN. Adolescent maturity and the brain: the promise and pitfalls of neuroscience research in adolescent health policy. J Adolesc Health. 2009;45(3):216-21. PubMed PMID: 19699416; PubMed Central PMCID: 2892678. FREE

231. Arain M, Haque M, Johal L, Mathur P, Nel W, Rais A, et al. Maturation of the adolescent brain. Neuropsychiatr Dis Treat. 2013;9:449-61. PubMed PMID: 23579318; PubMed Central PMCID: 3621648. FREE

235. Synaptogenesis Wikipedia [5-8-20]. Available from: https://en.wikipedia.org/wiki/Synaptogenesis.

236. Huttenlocher PR, Dabholkar AS. Regional differences in synaptogenesis in human cerebral cortex. J Comp Neurol. 1997;387(2):167-78. PubMed PMID: 9336221.

237. Jan YN, Jan LY. Branching out: mechanisms of dendritic arborization. Nat Rev Neurosci. 2010;11(5):316-28. PubMed PMID: 20404840; PubMed Central PMCID: 3079328. FREE

238. Synaptic Pruning New Scientist [5-6-20]. Available from: https://www.newscientist.com/article/dn20803-brains-synaptic-pruning-continues-into-your-20s/.

239. MRI Mayo Clinic [5-9-20]. Available from: https://www.mayoclinic.org/tests-procedures/mri/about/pac-20384768.

240. CT Scan Mayo Clinic [5-9-20]. Available from: https://www.mayoclinic.org/tests-procedures/ct-scan/about/pac-20393675.

241. fMRI Wikipedia [5-9-20]. Available from: https://en.wikipedia.org/wiki/Functional_magnetic_resonance_imaging.

242. Bloomfield MAP, Hindocha C, Green SF, Wall MB, Lees R, Petrilli K, et al. The neuropsychopharmacology of cannabis: A review of human imaging studies. Pharmacol Ther. 2019;195:132-61. PubMed PMID: 30347211; PubMed Central PMCID: 6416743. FREE

243. Blest-Hopley G, Giampietro V, Bhattacharyya S. Residual effects of cannabis use in adolescent and adult brains – A meta-analysis of fMRI studies. Neurosci Biobehav Rev. 2018;88:26-41. PubMed PMID: 29535069.

244. Ashtari M, Avants B, Cyckowski L, Cervellione KL, Roofeh D, Cook P, et al. Medial temporal structures and memory functions in adolescents with heavy cannabis use. J Psychiatr Res. 2011;45(8):1055-66. PubMed PMID: 21296361; PubMed Central PMCID: 3303223. FREE

245. Demirakca T, Sartorius A, Ende G, Meyer N, Welzel H, Skopp G, et al. Diminished gray matter in the hippocampus of cannabis users: possible protective effects of cannabidiol. Drug Alcohol Depend. 2011;114(2-3):242-5. PubMed PMID: 21050680.

246. Filbey FM, McQueeny T, Kadamangudi S, Bice C, Ketcherside A. Combined effects of marijuana and nicotine on memory performance and hippocampal volume. Behav Brain Res. 2015;293:46-53. PubMed PMID: 26187691; PubMed Central PMCID: 4567389. FREE

247. Lorenzetti V, Solowij N, Whittle S, Fornito A, Lubman DI, Pantelis C, et al. Gross morphological brain changes with chronic, heavy cannabis use. Br J Psychiatry. 2015;206(1):77-8. PubMed PMID: 25431432.

248. Matochik JA, Eldreth DA, Cadet JL, Bolla KI. Altered brain tissue composition in heavy marijuana users. Drug Alcohol Depend. 2005;77(1):23-30. PubMed PMID: 15607838.

249. Yucel M, Solowij N, Respondek C, Whittle S, Fornito A, Pantelis C, et al. Regional brain abnormalities associated with long-term heavy cannabis use. Arch Gen Psychiatry. 2008;65(6):694-701. PubMed PMID: 18519827.

250. Price JS, McQueeny T, Shollenbarger S, Browning EL, Wieser J, Lisdahl KM. Effects of marijuana use on prefrontal and parietal volumes and cognition in emerging adults. Psychopharmacology (Berl). 2015;232(16):2939-50. PubMed PMID: 25921032; PubMed Central PMCID: 4533900. FREE

251. Inferior Parietal Lobule Wikipedia [9/12/2020]. Available from: https://en.wikipedia.org/wiki/Inferior_parietal_lobule.

252. Rocchetti M, Crescini A, Borgwardt S, Caverzasi E, Politi P, Atakan Z, et al. Is cannabis neurotoxic for the healthy brain? A meta-analytical review of structural brain alterations in non-psychotic users. Psychiatry Clin Neurosci. 2013;67(7):483-92. PubMed PMID: 24118193. FREE

253. Chye Y, Suo C, Lorenzetti V, Batalla A, Cousijn J, Goudriaan AE, et al. Cortical surface morphology in long-term cannabis users: A multi-site MRI study. Eur Neuropsychopharmacol. 2019;29(2):257-65. PubMed PMID: 30558823.

254. D'Souza DC, Radhakrishnan R, Naganawa M, Ganesh S, Nabulsi N, Najafzadeh S, et al. Preliminary in vivo evidence of lower hippocampal synaptic density in cannabis use disorder. Mol Psychiatry. 2020. PubMed PMID: 32973170.

255. Executive function Wikipedia [4-17-20]. Available from: https://en.wikipedia.org/wiki/Executive_functions.

256. Broyd SJ, van Hell HH, Beale C, Yucel M, Solowij N. Acute and Chronic Effects of Cannabinoids on Human Cognition-A Systematic Review. Biol Psychiatry. 2016;79(7):557-67.. PubMed PMID: 26858214.

257. Cognition Wikipedia [4-15-20]. Available from: https://en.wikipedia.org/wiki/Cognition.

258. Greenwood PM, Parasuraman R. Neuronal and cognitive plasticity: a neurocognitive framework for ameliorating cognitive aging. Front Aging Neurosci. 2010;2:150. PubMed PMID: 21151819; PubMed Central PMCID: 2999838. FREE

259. Fernandes RM, Correa MG, Dos Santos MAR, Almeida A, Fagundes NCF, Maia LC, et al. The Effects of Moderate Physical Exercise on Adult Cognition: A Systematic Review. Front Physiol. 2018;9:667. PubMed PMID: 29937732; PubMed Central PMCID: 6002532. FREE

260. Kokubun K, Nemoto K, Yamakawa Y. Fish Intake May Affect Brain Structure and Improve Cognitive Ability in Healthy People. Front Aging Neurosci. 2020;12:76. PubMed PMID: 32265686; PubMed Central PMCID: 7103640. FREE

261. Rogge AK, Roder B, Zech A, Nagel V, Hollander K, Braumann KM, et al. Balance training improves memory and spatial cognition in healthy adults. Sci

Rep. 2017;7(1):5661. PubMed PMID: 28720898; PubMed Central PMCID: 5515881. FREE

262. Haskell-Ramsay CF, Jackson PA, Forster JS, Dodd FL, Bowerbank SL, Kennedy DO. The Acute Effects of Caffeinated Black Coffee on Cognition and Mood in Healthy Young and Older Adults. Nutrients. 2018;10(10). PubMed PMID: 30274327; PubMed Central PMCID: 6213082. FREE

263. Kinsella GJ, Pike KE, Wright BJ. Who benefits from cognitive intervention in older age? The role of executive function. Clin Neuropsychol. 2020:1-19. PubMed PMID: 32283994.

264. Klimova B, Valis M, Kuca K. Cognitive decline in normal aging and its prevention: a review on non-pharmacological lifestyle strategies. Clin Interv Aging. 2017;12:903-10. PubMed PMID: 28579767; PubMed Central PMCID: 5448694. FREE

265. Mende MA. Alcohol in the Aging Brain – The Interplay Between Alcohol Consumption, Cognitive Decline and the Cardiovascular System. Front Neurosci. 2019;13:713. PubMed PMID: 31333411; PubMed Central PMCID: 6624477. FREE

266. Kulick ER, Wellenius GA, Boehme AK, Joyce NR, Schupf N, Kaufman JD, et al. Long-term exposure to air pollution and trajectories of cognitive decline among older adults. Neurology. 2020. PubMed PMID: 32269113.

267. Armstrong NM, Bangen KJ, Au R, Gross AL. Associations Between Midlife (but Not Late-Life) Elevated Coronary Heart Disease Risk and Lower Cognitive Performance: Results From the Framingham Offspring Study. Am J Epidemiol. 2019;188(12):2175-87. PubMed PMID: 31576397; PubMed Central PMCID: 7036653. FREE

268. Levine DA, Gross AL, Briceno EM, Tilton N, Kabeto MU, Hingtgen SM, et al. Association Between Blood Pressure and Later-Life Cognition Among Black and White Individuals. JAMA Neurol. 2020. PubMed PMID: 32282019.

269. Andreotti C, Root JC, Ahles TA, McEwen BS, Compas BE. Cancer, coping, and cognition: a model for the role of stress reactivity in cancer-related cognitive decline. Psychooncology. 2015;24(6):617-23. PubMed PMID: 25286084; PubMed Central PMCID: 4387099. FREE

270. Hirsiger S, Hanggi J, Germann J, Vonmoos M, Preller KH, Engeli EJE, et al. Longitudinal changes in cocaine intake and cognition are linked to cortical thickness adaptations in cocaine users. Neuroimage Clin. 2019;21:101652. PubMed PMID: 30639181; PubMed Central PMCID: 6412021. FREE

271. Solowij N, Stephens RS, Roffman RA, Babor T, Kadden R, Miller M, et al. Cognitive functioning of long-term heavy cannabis users seeking treatment. JAMA. 2002;287(9):1123-31. PubMed PMID: 11879109.

272. Colizzi M, Tosato S, Ruggeri M. Cannabis and Cognition: Connecting the Dots towards the Understanding of the Relationship. Brain Sci. 2020;10(3). PubMed PMID: 32120842; PubMed Central PMCID: 7139821. FREE

273. Scott JC, Slomiak ST, Jones JD, Rosen AFG, Moore TM, Gur RC. Association of Cannabis With Cognitive Functioning in Adolescents and Young Adults: A Systematic Review and Meta-analysis. JAMA Psychiatry. 2018;75(6):585-95. PubMed PMID: 29710074; PubMed Central PMCID: 6137521. FREE

274. Becker MP, Collins PF, Schultz A, Urosevic S, Schmaling B, Luciana M. Longitudinal changes in cognition in

young adult cannabis users. J Clin Exp Neuropsychol. 2018;40(6):529-43. PubMed PMID: 29058519; PubMed Central PMCID: 6130912. FREE

275. Pope HG, Jr., Gruber AJ, Hudson JI, Huestis MA, Yurgelun-Todd D. Neuropsychological performance in long-term cannabis users. Arch Gen Psychiatry. 2001;58(10):909-15. PubMed PMID: 11576028.

276. Krzyzanowski DJ, Purdon SE. Duration of abstinence from cannabis is positively associated with verbal learning performance: A systematic review and meta-analysis. Neuropsychology. 2020;34(3):359-72. PubMed PMID: 31886689.

277. Paige KJ, Colder CR. Long-Term Effects of Early Adolescent Marijuana Use on Attentional and Inhibitory Control. J Stud Alcohol Drugs. 2020;81(2):164-72. PubMed PMID: 32359045.

278. Matheson J, Mann RE, Sproule B, Huestis MA, Wickens CM, Stoduto G, et al. Acute and residual mood and cognitive performance of young adults following smoked cannabis. Pharmacol Biochem Behav. 2020:172937. PubMed PMID: 32360692.

279. Wallace AL, Wade NE, Lisdahl KM. Impact of 2 Weeks of Monitored Abstinence on Cognition in Adolescent and Young Adult Cannabis Users. J Int Neuropsychol Soc. 2020:1-9. PubMed PMID: 32307027.

280. Crean RD, Tapert SF, Minassian A, Macdonald K, Crane NA, Mason BJ. Effects of chronic, heavy cannabis use on executive functions. J Addict Med. 2011;5(1):9-15. PubMed PMID: 21643485; PubMed Central PMCID: 3106308. FREE

281. Chung T, Bae SW, Mun EY, Suffoletto B, Nishiyama Y, Jang S, et al. Mobile Assessment of Acute Effects of Marijuana on Cognitive Functioning in Young Adults: Observational Study. JMIR Mhealth Uhealth. 2020;8(3):e16240. PubMed PMID: 32154789; PubMed Central PMCID: 7093776. FREE

282. Aloi J, Blair KS, Meffert H, White SF, Hwang S, Tyler PM, et al. Alcohol use disorder and cannabis use disorder symptomatology in adolescents is associated with dysfunction in neural processing of future events. Addict Biol. 2020:e12885. PubMed PMID: 32135572.

283. Bossong MG, Jager G, Bhattacharyya S, Allen P. Acute and non-acute effects of cannabis on human memory function: a critical review of neuroimaging studies. Curr Pharm Des. 2014;20(13):2114-25. PubMed PMID: 23829369.

284. McKetin R, Parasu P, Cherbuin N, Eramudugolla R, Anstey KJ. A longitudinal examination of the relationship between cannabis use and cognitive function in mid-life adults. Drug Alcohol Depend. 2016;169:134-40. PubMed PMID: 27810656.

285. Benitez A, Lauzon S, Nietert PJ, McRae-Clark A, Sherman BJ. Self-reported cognition and marijuana use in older adults: Results from the national epidemiologic survey on alcohol and related conditions-III. Addict Behav. 2020;108:106437. PubMed PMID: 32330763.

286. Rice J, Cameron M. Cannabinoids for Treatment of MS Symptoms: State of the Evidence. Curr Neurol Neurosci Rep. 2018;18(8):50. PubMed PMID: 29923025.

287. Rudroff T. Cannabis for Neuropathic Pain in Multiple Sclerosis-High Expectations, Poor Data. Front

Pharmacol. 2019;10:1239. PubMed PMID: 31695613; PubMed Central PMCID: 6817484. FREE

288. Honarmand K, Tierney MC, O'Connor P, Feinstein A. Effects of cannabis on cognitive function in patients with multiple sclerosis. Neurology. 2011;76(13):1153-60. PubMed PMID: 21444900; PubMed Central PMCID: 3068013. FREE

289. Feinstein A, Meza C, Stefan C, Staines RW. Coming off cannabis: a cognitive and magnetic resonance imaging study in patients with multiple sclerosis. Brain. 2019;142(9):2800-12. PubMed PMID: 31363742.

290. Feinstein A, Meza C, Stefan C, Staines WR. Discontinuing cannabis improves depression in people with multiple sclerosis: A short report. Mult Scler. 2020:1352458520934070. PubMed PMID: 32589554.

291. Tao C, Simpson S, Jr., Taylor BV, Blizzard L, Lucas RM, Ponsonby AL, et al. Onset Symptoms, Tobacco Smoking, and Progressive-Onset Phenotype Are Associated With a Delayed Onset of Multiple Sclerosis, and Marijuana Use With an Earlier Onset. Front Neurol. 2018;9:418. PubMed PMID: 29937751; PubMed Central PMCID: 6003245. FREE

292. Ghaffar O, Feinstein A. Multiple sclerosis and cannabis: a cognitive and psychiatric study. Neurology. 2008;71(3):164-9. PubMed PMID: 18272863.

293. Papathanasopoulos P, Messinis L, Lyros E, Kastellakis A, Panagis G. Multiple sclerosis, cannabinoids, and cognition. J Neuropsychiatry Clin Neurosci. 2008;20(1):36-51. PubMed PMID: 18305283.

294. Patel VP, Feinstein A. Cannabis and cognitive functioning in multiple sclerosis: The role

of gender. Mult Scler J Exp Transl Clin. 2017;3(2):2055217317713027. PubMed PMID: 28634543; PubMed Central PMCID: 5468765. FREE

295. Romero K, Pavisian B, Staines WR, Feinstein A. Multiple sclerosis, cannabis, and cognition: A structural MRI study. Neuroimage Clin. 2015;8:140-7. PubMed PMID: 26106538; PubMed Central PMCID: 4473732. FREE

296. Penner IK, Hartung HP. The dark side of the moon: looking beyond beneficial effects of cannabis use in multiple sclerosis. Brain. 2019;142(9):2552-5. PubMed PMID: 31497861.

297. Memory Wikipedia [4-19-20]. Available from: https://en.wikipedia.org/wiki/Memory.

298. Long Term Memory Wikipedia [4-19-20]. Available from: https://en.wikipedia.org/wiki/Long-term_memory.

299. Schuster RM, Gilman J, Schoenfeld D, Evenden J, Hareli M, Ulysse C, et al. One Month of Cannabis Abstinence in Adolescents and Young Adults Is Associated With Improved Memory. J Clin Psychiatry. 2018;79(6). PubMed PMID: 30408351; PubMed Central PMCID: 6587572. FREE

300. Adam KCS, Doss MK, Pabon E, Vogel EK, de Wit H. Delta(9)-Tetrahydrocannabinol (THC) impairs visual working memory performance: a randomized crossover trial. Neuropsychopharmacology. 2020. PubMed PMID: 32386395.

301. fMRI Wikipedia [4-19-20]. Available from: https://en.wikipedia.org/wiki/Functional_magnetic_resonance_imaging.

302. Cousijn J, Vingerhoets WA, Koenders L, de Haan L, van den Brink W, Wiers RW, et al. Relationship between working-memory network function and substance use: a 3-year longitudinal fMRI study in heavy cannabis users and controls. Addict Biol. 2014;19(2):282-93. PubMed PMID: 24589297.

303. Cousijn J, Wiers RW, Ridderinkhof KR, van den Brink W, Veltman DJ, Goudriaan AE. Effect of baseline cannabis use and working-memory network function on changes in cannabis use in heavy cannabis users: a prospective fMRI study. Hum Brain Mapp. 2014;35(5):2470-82. PubMed PMID: 24038570.

304. Schweinsburg AD, Schweinsburg BC, Medina KL, McQueeny T, Brown SA, Tapert SF. The influence of recency of use on fMRI response during spatial working memory in adolescent marijuana users. J Psychoactive Drugs. 2010;42(3):401-12. PubMed PMID: 21053763; PubMed Central PMCID: 3016644. FREE

305. Jacobsen LK, Mencl WE, Westerveld M, Pugh KR. Impact of cannabis use on brain function in adolescents. Ann N Y Acad Sci. 2004;1021:384-90. PubMed PMID: 15251914.

306. Schweinsburg AD, Nagel BJ, Schweinsburg BC, Park A, Theilmann RJ, Tapert SF. Abstinent adolescent marijuana users show altered fMRI response during spatial working memory. Psychiatry Res. 2008;163(1):40-51. PubMed PMID: 18356027; PubMed Central PMCID: 2832586. FREE

307. Becker B, Wagner D, Gouzoulis-Mayfrank E, Spuentrup E, Daumann J. The impact of early-onset cannabis use on functional brain correlates of working memory. Prog Neuropsychopharmacol Biol Psychiatry. 2010;34(6):837-45. PubMed PMID: 20363277.

308. Kanayama G, Rogowska J, Pope HG, Gruber SA, Yurgelun-Todd DA. Spatial working memory in heavy cannabis users: a functional magnetic resonance imaging study. Psychopharmacology (Berl). 2004;176(3-4):239-47. PubMed PMID: 15205869.

309. Padula CB, Schweinsburg AD, Tapert SF. Spatial working memory performance and fMRI activation interaction in abstinent adolescent marijuana users. Psychol Addict Behav. 2007;21(4):478-87. PubMed PMID: 18072830; PubMed Central PMCID: 2373252. FREE

310. Jager G, Block RI, Luijten M, Ramsey NF. Cannabis use and memory brain function in adolescent boys: a cross-sectional multicenter functional magnetic resonance imaging study. J Am Acad Child Adolesc Psychiatry. 2010;49(6):561-72, 72 e1-3. PubMed PMID: 20494266; PubMed Central PMCID: 2918244. FREE

311. Smith AM, Longo CA, Fried PA, Hogan MJ, Cameron I. Effects of marijuana on visuospatial working memory: an fMRI study in young adults. Psychopharmacology (Berl). 2010;210(3):429-38. PubMed PMID: 20401748.

312. Becker B, Wagner D, Gouzoulis-Mayfrank E, Spuentrup E, Daumann J. Altered parahippocampal functioning in cannabis users is related to the frequency of use. Psychopharmacology (Berl). 2010;209(4):361-74. PubMed PMID: 20300735.

313. Olla P, Rykulski N, Hurtubise JL, Bartol S, Foote R, Cutler L, et al. Short-term effects of cannabis consumption on cognitive performance in medical cannabis patients. Appl Neuropsychol Adult. 2019:1-11. PubMed PMID: 31790276.

314. Marijuana improves memory in old mice. Nature. 2017;545(7653):137. PubMed PMID: 32076258.

315. Bilkei-Gorzo A, Albayram O, Draffehn A, Michel K, Piyanova A, Oppenheimer H, et al. A chronic low dose of Delta(9)-tetrahydrocannabinol (THC) restores cognitive function in old mice. Nat Med. 2017;23(6):782-7. PubMed PMID: 28481360.

316. Sarne Y, Toledano R, Rachmany L, Sasson E, Doron R. Reversal of age-related cognitive impairments in mice by an extremely low dose of tetrahydrocannabinol. Neurobiol Aging. 2018;61:177-86. PubMed PMID: 29107185.

317. Doss MK, Weafer J, Gallo DA, de Wit H. Delta(9)-Tetrahydrocannabinol at Retrieval Drives False Recollection of Neutral and Emotional Memories. Biol Psychiatry. 2018;84(10):743-50. PubMed PMID: 29884456.

318. Mercuri K, Terrett G, Henry JD, Curran HV, Elliott M, Rendell PG. Episodic foresight deficits in regular, but not recreational, cannabis users. J Psychopharmacol. 2018;32(8):876-82. PubMed PMID: 29897004.

319. Braidwood R, Mansell S, Waldron J, Rendell PG, Kamboj SK, Curran HV. Non-Dependent and Dependent Daily Cannabis Users Differ in Mental Health but Not Prospective Memory Ability. Front Psychiatry. 2018;9:97. PubMed PMID: 29636705; PubMed Central PMCID: 5880932. FREE

320. Montgomery C, Seddon AL, Fisk JE, Murphy PN, Jansari A. Cannabis-related deficits in real-world memory. Hum Psychopharmacol. 2012;27(2):217-25. PubMed PMID: 22389086.

321. False Memories_The Scientist [5-8-20]. Available from: The Scientist May 1, 2020

322. Kloft L, Otgaar H, Blokland A, Garbaciak A, Monds LA, Ramaekers JG. False memory formation in cannabis users: a field study. Psychopharmacology (Berl). 2019;236(12):3439-50. PubMed PMID: 31250074; PubMed Central PMCID: 6892757. FREE

323. Riba J, Valle M, Sampedro F, Rodriguez-Pujadas A, Martinez-Horta S, Kulisevsky J, et al. Telling true from false: cannabis users show increased susceptibility to false memories. Mol Psychiatry. 2015;20(6):772-7. PubMed PMID: 25824306; PubMed Central PMCID: 4441258. FREE

324. Evans J.R. SCN, Russano M.B. Intoxicated witnesses and suspects: Procedures and prevalence according to law enforcement. Psychol Public Policy Law. 2009;15:194–221.

325. Flowe H.D. CMF, Kloft L., Jores T., Stevens L.M. Impact of alcohol and other drugs on eyewitness memory. In: R. Bull IB-G, editor. The Routledge International Handbook of Legal and Investigative Psychology. London, UK: Routledge; 2020. p. 149–62.

326. Kloft L, Otgaar H, Blokland A, Monds LA, Toennes SW, Loftus EF, et al. Cannabis increases susceptibility to false memory. Proc Natl Acad Sci U S A. 2020;117(9):4585-9. PubMed PMID: 32041881; PubMed Central PMCID: 7060677. FREE

327. Intelligence Quotient Wikipedia [4-28-20]. Available from: https://en.wikipedia.org/wiki/Intelligence_quotient.

328. Fried P, Watkinson B, James D, Gray R. Current and former marijuana use: preliminary findings of a longitudinal study of effects on IQ in young adults.

CMAJ. 2002;166(7):887-91. PubMed PMID: 11949984; PubMed Central PMCID: 100921. FREE

329. Meier MH, Caspi A, Ambler A, Harrington H, Houts R, Keefe RS, et al. Persistent cannabis users show neuropsychological decline from childhood to midlife. Proc Natl Acad Sci U S A. 2012;109(40):E2657-64. PubMed PMID: 22927402; PubMed Central PMCID: 3479587. FREE

330. Pope HG, Jr., Gruber AJ, Hudson JI, Cohane G, Huestis MA, Yurgelun-Todd D. Early-onset cannabis use and cognitive deficits: what is the nature of the association? Drug Alcohol Depend. 2003;69(3):303-10. PubMed PMID: 12633916.

331. Goldschmidt L, Richardson GA, Willford J, Day NL. Prenatal marijuana exposure and intelligence test performance at age 6. J Am Acad Child Adolesc Psychiatry. 2008;47(3):254-63. PubMed PMID: 18216735.

332. Mokrysz C, Landy R, Gage SH, Munafo MR, Roiser JP, Curran HV. Are IQ and educational outcomes in teenagers related to their cannabis use? A prospective cohort study. J Psychopharmacol. 2016;30(2):159-68. PubMed PMID: 26739345; PubMed Central PMCID: 4724860. FREE

333 Jackson NJ, Isen JD, Khoddam R, Irons D, Tuvblad C, Iacono WG, et al. Impact of adolescent marijuana use on intelligence: Results from two longitudinal twin studies. Proc Natl Acad Sci U S A. 2016;113(5):E500-8. PubMed PMID: 26787878; PubMed Central PMCID: 4747759. FREE

334. Silveira MM, Adams WK, Morena M, Hill MN, Winstanley CA. Delta(9)-Tetrahydrocannabinol decreases willingness to exert cognitive effort in

male rats. J Psychiatry Neurosci. 2017;42(2):131-8. PubMed PMID: 28245177; PubMed Central PMCID: 5373702. FREE

335. Zamberletti E, Gabaglio M, Prini P, Rubino T, Parolaro D. Cortical neuroinflammation contributes to long-term cognitive dysfunctions following adolescent delta-9-tetrahydrocannabinol treatment in female rats. Eur Neuropsychopharmacol. 2015;25(12):2404-15. PubMed PMID: 26499171.

336. Panlilio LV, Ferre S, Yasar S, Thorndike EB, Schindler CW, Goldberg SR. Combined effects of THC and caffeine on working memory in rats. Br J Pharmacol. 2012;165(8):2529-38. PubMed PMID: 21699509; PubMed Central PMCID: 3423236. FREE

337. Moore NL, Greenleaf AL, Acheson SK, Wilson WA, Swartzwelder HS, Kuhn CM. Role of cannabinoid receptor type 1 desensitization in greater tetrahydrocannabinol impairment of memory in adolescent rats. J Pharmacol Exp Ther. 2010;335(2):294-301. PubMed PMID: 20668056; PubMed Central PMCID: 2967405. FREE

338. Rubino T, Realini N, Braida D, Alberio T, Capurro V, Vigano D, et al. The depressive phenotype induced in adult female rats by adolescent exposure to THC is associated with cognitive impairment and altered neuroplasticity in the prefrontal cortex. Neurotox Res. 2009;15(4):291-302. PubMed PMID: 19384563.

339. Senn R, Keren O, Hefetz A, Sarne Y. Long-term cognitive deficits induced by a single, extremely low dose of tetrahydrocannabinol (THC): behavioral, pharmacological and biochemical studies in mice.

Pharmacol Biochem Behav. 2008;88(3):230-7. PubMed PMID: 17888506.

340. Niyuhire F, Varvel SA, Martin BR, Lichtman AH. Exposure to marijuana smoke impairs memory retrieval in mice. J Pharmacol Exp Ther. 2007;322(3):1067-75. PubMed PMID: 17586723.

341. Quinn HR, Matsumoto I, Callaghan PD, Long LE, Arnold JC, Gunasekaran N, et al. Adolescent rats find repeated Delta(9)-THC less aversive than adult rats but display greater residual cognitive deficits and changes in hippocampal protein expression following exposure. Neuropsychopharmacology. 2008;33(5):1113-26. PubMed PMID: 17581536.

342. Mishima K, Egashira N, Hirosawa N, Fujii M, Matsumoto Y, Iwasaki K, et al. Characteristics of learning and memory impairment induced by delta9-tetrahydrocannabinol in rats. Jpn J Pharmacol. 2001;87(4):297-308. PubMed PMID: 11829149.

343. Varvel SA, Hamm RJ, Martin BR, Lichtman AH. Differential effects of delta 9-THC on spatial reference and working memory in mice. Psychopharmacology (Berl). 2001;157(2):142-50. PubMed PMID: 11594438.

344. Verrico CD, Mathai DS, Gu H, Sampson AR, Lewis DA. Recovery from impaired working memory performance during chronic Delta-9-tetrahydrocannabinol administration to adolescent rhesus monkeys. J Psychopharmacol. 2020;34(2):211-20. PubMed PMID: 31621487.

345. Bruijnzeel AW, Knight P, Panunzio S, Xue S, Bruner MM, Wall SC, et al. Effects in rats of adolescent exposure to cannabis smoke or THC on emotional behavior and cognitive function in adulthood. Psychopharmacology

(Berl). 2019;236(9):2773-84. PubMed PMID: 31044291; PubMed Central PMCID: 6752736. FREE

346. Suliman NA, Taib CNM, Moklas MAM, Basir R. Delta-9-Tetrahydrocannabinol ((9)-THC) Induce Neurogenesis and Improve Cognitive Performances of Male Sprague Dawley Rats. Neurotox Res. 2018;33(2):402-11. PubMed PMID: 28933048; PubMed Central PMCID: 5766723. FREE

347. Murphy M, Mills S, Winstone J, Leishman E, Wager-Miller J, Bradshaw H, et al. Chronic Adolescent Delta(9)-Tetrahydrocannabinol Treatment of Male Mice Leads to Long-Term Cognitive and Behavioral Dysfunction, Which Are Prevented by Concurrent Cannabidiol Treatment. Cannabis Cannabinoid Res. 2017;2(1):235-46. PubMed PMID: 29098186; PubMed Central PMCID: 5655843. FREE

348. Brancato A, Castelli V, Lavanco G, Marino RAM, Cannizzaro C. In utero Delta9-tetrahydrocannabinol exposure confers vulnerability towards cognitive impairments and alcohol drinking in the adolescent offspring: Is there a role for neuropeptide Y? J Psychopharmacol. 2020:269881120916135. PubMed PMID: 32338122.

349. Berthoux C, Hamieh AM, Rogliardo A, Doucet EL, Coudert C, Ango F, et al. Early 5-HT6 receptor blockade prevents symptom onset in a model of adolescent cannabis abuse. EMBO Mol Med. 2020:e10605. PubMed PMID: 32329240.

Chapter 7: Cannabis and the Risk of Mental Illness: Refs. 350-431

Psychosis and Cannabis Induced Psychosis; Paranoia; Schizophrenia; The two biggest things about

Weed and Schizophrenia; The Chicken or the Egg problem; Depression, Anxiety and Bipolar Disorder, Distress Tolerance and Cannabis

350. Gage SH, Hickman M, Zammit S. Association Between Cannabis and Psychosis: Epidemiologic Evidence. Biol Psychiatry. 2016;79(7):549-56. PubMed PMID: 26386480.

351. Moore TH, Zammit S, Lingford-Hughes A, Barnes TR, Jones PB, Burke M, et al. Cannabis use and risk of psychotic or affective mental health outcomes: a systematic review. Lancet. 2007;370(9584):319-28. PubMed PMID: 17662880.

352. Sideli L, Quigley H, La Cascia C, Murray RM. Cannabis Use and the Risk of Psychosis and Affective Disorders. J Dual Diagn. 2019:1-21. PubMed PMID: 31647377.

353. Hall W, Degenhardt L. Cannabis use and the risk of developing a psychotic disorder. World Psychiatry. 2008;7(2):68-71. PubMed PMID: 18560513; PubMed Central PMCID: 2424288. FREE

354. Psychosis NIMH. Available from: https://www.nimh.nih.gov/health/topics/schizophrenia/raise/raise-questions-and-answers.shtml#1.

355. Psychosis Wikipedia. Available from: https://en.wikipedia.org/wiki/Psychosis.

356. Thomas H. Psychiatric symptoms in cannabis users. Br J Psychiatry. 1993;163:141-9. PubMed PMID: 8075903.

357. Shah D, Chand P, Bandawar M, Benegal V, Murthy P. Cannabis induced psychosis and subsequent psychiatric disorders. Asian J Psychiatr. 2017;30:180-4. PubMed PMID: 29096386.

358. Johns A. Psychiatric effects of cannabis. Br J Psychiatry. 2001;178:116-22. PubMed PMID: 11157424.

359. Ruby S. Grewal MD TPG, MD. Cannabis-Induced Psychosis: A Review Psychiatric times2017. Available from: https://www.psychiatrictimes.com/substance-use-disorder/cannabis-induced-psychosis-review.

360. Tunving K. Psychiatric effects of cannabis use. Acta Psychiatr Scand. 1985;72(3):209-17. PubMed PMID: 3000137.

361. Di Forti M, Quattrone D, Freeman TP, Tripoli G, Gayer-Anderson C, Quigley H, et al. The contribution of cannabis use to variation in the incidence of psychotic disorder across Europe (EU-GEI): a multicentre case-control study. Lancet Psychiatry. 2019;6(5):427-36. PubMed PMID: 30902669.

362. Gerlach J, Koret B, Geres N, Matic K, Prskalo-Cule D, Zadravec Vrbanc T, et al. Clinical Challenges in Patients with First Episode Psychosis and Cannabis Use: Mini-Review and a Case Study. Psychiatr Danub. 2019;31(Suppl 2):162-70. PubMed PMID: 31158117.

363. Arendt M, Rosenberg R, Foldager L, Perto G, Munk-Jorgensen P. Cannabis-induced psychosis and subsequent schizophrenia-spectrum disorders: follow-up study of 535 incident cases. Br J Psychiatry. 2005;187:510-5. PubMed PMID: 16319402.

364. Henquet C, Rosa A, Delespaul P, Papiol S, Fananas L, van Os J, et al. COMT ValMet moderation of cannabis-induced psychosis: a momentary assessment study of 'switching on' hallucinations in the flow of daily life. Acta Psychiatr Scand. 2009;119(2):156-60. PubMed PMID: 18808401.

365. Vaessen TSJ, de Jong L, Schafer AT, Damen T, Uittenboogaard A, Krolinski P, et al. The interaction between cannabis use and the Val158Met polymorphism of the COMT gene in psychosis: A transdiagnostic meta – analysis. PLoS One. 2018;13(2):e0192658. PubMed PMID: 29444152; PubMed Central PMCID: 5812637. FREE

367. Mane A, Berge D, Penzol MJ, Parellada M, Bioque M, Lobo A, et al. Cannabis use, COMT, BDNF and age at first-episode psychosis. Psychiatry Res. 2017;250:38-43. PubMed PMID: 28142064.

368. Murrie B, Lappin J, Large M, Sara G. Transition of Substance-Induced, Brief, and Atypical Psychoses to Schizophrenia: A Systematic Review and Meta-analysis. Schizophr Bull. 2019. PubMed PMID: 31618428.

369. Paranoia- Wikipedia [9/1/2020]. Available from: https://en.wikipedia.org/wiki/Paranoia.

370. Freeman D, McManus S, Brugha T, Meltzer H, Jenkins R, Bebbington P. Concomitants of paranoia in the general population. Psychol Med. 2011;41(5):923-36. PubMed PMID: 20735884.

371. Freeman D, Morrison PD, Murray RM, Evans N, Lister R, Dunn G. Persecutory ideation and a history of cannabis use. Schizophr Res. 2013;148(1-3):122-5. PubMed PMID: 23806582.

372. Coid JW, Ullrich S, Bebbington P, Fazel S, Keers R. Paranoid Ideation and Violence: Meta-analysis of Individual Subject Data of 7 Population Surveys. Schizophr Bull. 2016;42(4):907-15.. PubMed PMID: 26884548; PubMed Central PMCID: 4903063. FREE

373. Schizophrenia-Wikipedia [9/1/2020]. Available from: https://en.wikipedia.org/wiki/Schizophrenia.

374. Kendler KS, Ohlsson H, Sundquist J, Sundquist K. Prediction of Onset of Substance-Induced Psychotic Disorder and Its Progression to Schizophrenia in a Swedish National Sample. Am J Psychiatry. 2019;176(9):711-9. PubMed PMID: 31055966; PubMed Central PMCID: 6718312. FREE

375. Owen MJ, Sawa A, Mortensen PB. Schizophrenia. Lancet. 2016;388(10039):86-97. PubMed PMID: 26777917; PubMed Central PMCID: 4940219. FREE

376. Boksa P. Abnormal synaptic pruning in schizophrenia: Urban myth or reality? J Psychiatry Neurosci. 2012;37(2):75-7. PubMed PMID: 22339991; PubMed Central PMCID: 3297065. FREE

377. Blest-Hopley G, Colizzi M, Giampietro V, Bhattacharyya S. Is the Adolescent Brain at Greater Vulnerability to the Effects of Cannabis? A Narrative Review of the Evidence. Front Psychiatry. 2020;11:859. PubMed PMID: 33005157; PubMed Central PMCID: 7479242. FREE

378. Evensen S., Wisløff T., Lystad J.U. , Bull H., Ueland T., and Falkum E. Prevalence, Employment Rate, and Cost of Schizophrenia in a High-Income Welfare Society: A Population-Based Study Using Comprehensive Health and Welfare Registers. Schizophr Bull. 2016 Mar; 42(2): 476–483.PubMed PMID: 26433216 PubMed Central PMCID: 4753607 FREE

379. Andreasson S, Allebeck P, Engstrom A, Rydberg U. Cannabis and schizophrenia. A longitudinal study of Swedish conscripts. Lancet. 1987;2(8574):1483-6. PubMed PMID: 2892048.

380. Hjorthoj C, Albert N, Nordentoft M. Association of Substance Use Disorders With Conversion From Schizotypal Disorder to Schizophrenia. JAMA Psychiatry.

2018;75(7):733-9. PubMed PMID: 29710317; PubMed Central PMCID: 6145672. FREE

381. Khantzian EJ. The self-medication hypothesis of substance use disorders: a reconsideration and recent applications. Harv Rev Psychiatry. 1997;4(5):231-44. PubMed PMID: 9385000.

382 Kolliakou A, Joseph C, Ismail K, Atakan Z, Murray RM. Why do patients with psychosis use cannabis and are they ready to change their use? Int J Dev Neurosci. 2011;29(3):335-46. PubMed PMID: 21172414.

383. Hall W. Cannabis use and psychosis. Drug Alcohol Rev. 1998;17(4):433-44. PubMed PMID: 16203510.

384. Griffith-Lendering MF, Wigman JT, Prince van Leeuwen A, Huijbregts SC, Huizink AC, Ormel J, et al. Cannabis use and vulnerability for psychosis in early adolescence–a TRAILS study. Addiction. 2013;108(4):733-40. PubMed PMID: 23216690.

385. Arseneault L, Cannon M, Poulton R, Murray R, Caspi A, Moffitt TE. Cannabis use in adolescence and risk for adult psychosis: longitudinal prospective study. BMJ. 2002;325(7374):1212-3. PubMed PMID: 12446537; PubMed Central PMCID: 135493. FREE

386. Kuepper R, van Os J, Lieb R, Wittchen HU, Hofler M, Henquet C. Continued cannabis use and risk of incidence and persistence of psychotic symptoms: 10 year follow-up cohort study. BMJ. 2011;342:d738. PubMed PMID: 21363868; PubMed Central PMCID: 3047001. FREE

387. Bourque J, Afzali MH, Conrod PJ. Association of Cannabis Use With Adolescent Psychotic Symptoms.

JAMA Psychiatry. 2018;75(8):864-6. PubMed PMID: 29874357; PubMed Central PMCID: 6584279. FREE

388. Compton MT, Kelley ME, Ramsay CE, Pringle M, Goulding SM, Esterberg ML, et al. Association of pre-onset cannabis, alcohol, and tobacco use with age at onset of prodrome and age at onset of psychosis in first-episode patients. Am J Psychiatry. 2009;166(11):1251-7. PubMed PMID: 19797432; PubMed Central PMCID: 3662470. FREE

389. Neill E, Tan EJ, Toh WL, Selvendra A, Morgan VA, Rossell SL, et al. Examining which factors influence age of onset in males and females with schizophrenia. Schizophr Res. 2020. PubMed PMID: 32883558.

390. Gage SH, Jones HJ, Burgess S, Bowden J, Davey Smith G, Zammit S, et al. Assessing causality in associations between cannabis use and schizophrenia risk: a two-sample Mendelian randomization study. Psychol Med. 2017;47(5):971-80. PubMed PMID: 27928975; PubMed Central PMCID: 5341491. FREE

391. Clausen L, Hjorthoj CR, Thorup A, Jeppesen P, Petersen L, Bertelsen M, et al. Change in cannabis use, clinical symptoms and social functioning among patients with first-episode psychosis: a 5-year follow-up study of patients in the OPUS trial. Psychol Med. 2014;44(1):117-26. PubMed PMID: 23590927.

392. Schoeler T, Petros N, Di Forti M, Pingault JB, Klamerus E, Foglia E, et al. Association Between Continued Cannabis Use and Risk of Relapse in First-Episode Psychosis: A Quasi-Experimental Investigation Within an Observational Study. JAMA Psychiatry. 2016;73(11):1173-9. PubMed PMID: 27680429.

393. Hatzigiakoumis DS, Martinotti G, Giannantonio MD, Janiri L. Anhedonia and substance dependence: clinical correlates and treatment options. Front Psychiatry. 2011;2:10. PubMed PMID: 21556280; PubMed Central PMCID: 3089992. FREE

394. Gobbi G, Atkin T, Zytynski T, Wang S, Askari S, Boruff J, et al. Association of Cannabis Use in Adolescence and Risk of Depression, Anxiety, and Suicidality in Young Adulthood: A Systematic Review and Meta-analysis. JAMA Psychiatry. 2019;76(4):426-34. PubMed PMID: 30758486; PubMed Central PMCID: 6450286. FREE

395. Esmaeelzadeh S, Moraros J, Thorpe L, Bird Y. The association between depression, anxiety and substance use among Canadian post-secondary students. Neuropsychiatr Dis Treat. 2018;14:3241-51. PubMed PMID: 30538482; PubMed Central PMCID: 6260190. FREE

396. Horwood LJ, Fergusson DM, Coffey C, Patton GC, Tait R, Smart D, et al. Cannabis and depression: an integrative data analysis of four Australasian cohorts. Drug Alcohol Depend. 2012;126(3):369-78. PubMed PMID: 22749560.

397. Lev-Ran S, Roerecke M, Le Foll B, George TP, McKenzie K, Rehm J. The association between cannabis use and depression: a systematic review and meta-analysis of longitudinal studies. Psychol Med. 2014;44(4):797-810. PubMed PMID: 23795762.

398. Gukasyan N, Strain EC. Relationship between cannabis use frequency and major depressive disorder in adolescents: Findings from the National Survey on Drug Use and Health 2012-2017. Drug Alcohol Depend.

2020;208:107867. PubMed PMID: 31958677; PubMed Central PMCID: 7039755. FREE

3929 Van Ameringen M, Zhang J, Patterson B, Turna J. The role of cannabis in treating anxiety: an update. Curr Opin Psychiatry. 2020;33(1):1-7. PubMed PMID: 31688192.

400. Volkow ND, Hampson AJ, Baler RD. Don't Worry, Be Happy: Endocannabinoids and Cannabis at the Intersection of Stress and Reward. Annu Rev Pharmacol Toxicol. 2017;57:285-308. PubMed PMID: 27618739.

401. Anxiety Anxiety.org [9/11/2020]. Available from: https://www.anxiety.org/what-is-anxiety.

402. NAMI Anxiety Disorders [9/11/2020]. Available from: https://www.nami.org/About-Mental-Illness/Mental-Health-Conditions/Anxiety-Disorders.

403. Anxiety disorders Mayo Clinic [9/11/2020]. Available from: https://www.mayoclinic.org/diseases-conditions/anxiety/symptoms-causes/syc-20350961.

404 Turna J, Patterson B, Van Ameringen M. Is cannabis treatment for anxiety, mood, and related disorders ready for prime time? Depress Anxiety. 2017;34(11):1006-17. PubMed PMID: 28636769.

405. Bonini SA, Premoli M, Tambaro S, Kumar A, Maccarinelli G, Memo M, et al. Cannabis sativa: A comprehensive ethnopharmacological review of a medicinal plant with a long history. J Ethnopharmacol. 2018;227:300-15. PubMed PMID: 30205181.

406. Ramikie TS, Patel S. Endocannabinoid signaling in the amygdala: anatomy, synaptic signaling, behavior, and adaptations to stress. Neuroscience. 2012;204:38-52.

. PubMed PMID: 21884761; PubMed Central PMCID: 3236282. FREE

407. Masataka N. Anxiolytic Effects of Repeated Cannabidiol Treatment in Teenagers With Social Anxiety Disorders. Front Psychol. 2019;10:2466. PubMed PMID: 31787910; PubMed Central PMCID: 6856203. FREE

408. Lim K, See YM, Lee J. A Systematic Review of the Effectiveness of Medical Cannabis for Psychiatric, Movement and Neurodegenerative Disorders. Clin Psychopharmacol Neurosci. 2017;15(4):301-12. PubMed PMID: 29073741; PubMed Central PMCID: 5678490. FREE

409. Childs E, Lutz JA, de Wit H. Dose-related effects of delta-9-THC on emotional responses to acute psychosocial stress. Drug Alcohol Depend. 2017;177:136-44. PubMed PMID: 28599212; PubMed Central PMCID: 6349031. FREE

410. Bossong MG, Jansma JM, van Hell HH, Jager G, Kahn RS, Ramsey NF. Default mode network in the effects of Delta9-Tetrahydrocannabinol (THC) on human executive function. PLoS One. 2013;8(7):e70074. PubMed PMID: 23936144; PubMed Central PMCID: 3729458. FREE

411. Fusar-Poli P, Allen P, Bhattacharyya S, Crippa JA, Mechelli A, Borgwardt S, et al. Modulation of effective connectivity during emotional processing by Delta 9-tetrahydrocannabinol and cannabidiol. Int J Neuropsychopharmacol. 2010;13(4):421-32. PubMed PMID: 19775500.

412. Feingold D, Weiser M, Rehm J, Lev-Ran S. The association between cannabis use and anxiety disorders: Results from a population-based representative sample.

Eur Neuropsychopharmacol. 2016;26(3):493-505. PubMed PMID: 26775742.

413. Degenhardt L, Coffey C, Romaniuk H, Swift W, Carlin JB, Hall WD, et al. The persistence of the association between adolescent cannabis use and common mental disorders into young adulthood. Addiction. 2013;108(1):124-33. PubMed PMID: 22775447.

414. Hall W, Solowij N. Adverse effects of cannabis. Lancet. 1998;352(9140):1611-6. PubMed PMID: 9843121.

410. Roy-Byrne PP, Uhde TW. Exogenous factors in panic disorder: clinical and research implications. J Clin Psychiatry. 1988;49(2):56-61. PubMed PMID: 3276668.

415. Tournier M, Sorbara F, Gindre C, Swendsen JD, Verdoux H. Cannabis use and anxiety in daily life: a naturalistic investigation in a non-clinical population. Psychiatry Res. 2003;118(1):1-8. PubMed PMID: 12759155.

416. Hollister LE. Health aspects of cannabis. Pharmacol Rev. 1986;38(1):1-20. Epub 1986/03/01. PubMed PMID: 3520605.

417. Smaga I, Bystrowska B, Gawlinski D, Przegalinski E, Filip M. The endocannabinoid/endovanilloid system and depression. Curr Neuropharmacol. 2014;12(5):462-74. PubMed PMID: 25426013; PubMed Central PMCID: 4243035. FREE

418. Hirvonen J, Goodwin RS, Li CT, Terry GE, Zoghbi SS, Morse C, et al. Reversible and regionally selective downregulation of brain cannabinoid CB1 receptors in chronic daily cannabis smokers. Mol Psychiatry. 2012;17(6):642-9. PubMed PMID: 21747398; PubMed Central PMCID: 3223558. FREE

419. Suplita RL, 2nd, Eisenstein SA, Neely MH, Moise AM, Hohmann AG. Cross-sensitization and cross-tolerance between exogenous cannabinoid antinociception and endocannabinoid-mediated stress-induced analgesia. Neuropharmacology. 2008;54(1):161-71.PubMed PMID: 17714742; PubMed Central PMCID: 2771679. FREE

420. Mayer TA, Matar MA, Kaplan Z, Zohar J, Cohen H. Blunting of the HPA-axis underlies the lack of preventive efficacy of early post-stressor single-dose Delta-9-tetrahydrocannabinol (THC). Pharmacol Biochem Behav. 2014;122:307-18. PubMed PMID: 24814135.

421. Beyer CE, Dwyer JM, Piesla MJ, Platt BJ, Shen R, Rahman Z, et al. Depression-like phenotype following chronic CB1 receptor antagonism. Neurobiol Dis. 2010;39(2):148-55. PubMed PMID: 20381618.

422. Kedzior KK, Laeber LT. A positive association between anxiety disorders and cannabis use or cannabis use disorders in the general population–a meta-analysis of 31 studies. BMC Psychiatry. 2014;14:136. PubMed PMID: 24884989; PubMed Central PMCID: 4032500. FREE

423. Distress Tolerance-Very Well MInd [8/20/20]. Available from: https://www.verywellmind. com/distress-tolerance-2797294.

424. Distress Tolerance- Wikipedia [8/20-2020]. Available from: https://en.wikipedia.org/wiki/Distress_tolerance.

425. Peraza N, Smit T, Garey L, Manning K, Buckner JD, Zvolensky MJ. Distress tolerance and cessation-related cannabis processes: The role of cannabis use coping motives. Addict Behav. 2019;90:164-70. PubMed PMID: 30408699.

426. Dialectic Behaviour Therapy- Wikipedia [8/20/2020]. Available from: https://en.wikipedia.org/wiki/Dialectical_behavior_therapy.

427. Dimeff LA, Linehan MM. Dialectical behavior therapy for substance abusers. Addict Sci Clin Pract. 2008;4(2):39-47. PubMed PMID: 18497717; PubMed Central PMCID: 2797106. FREE

428. Bipolar Disorder-Mayo Clinic [8/21/2020]. Available from: https://www.mayoclinic.org/diseases-conditions/bipolar-disorder/symptoms-causes/syc-20355955.

429. Gibbs M, Winsper C, Marwaha S, Gilbert E, Broome M, Singh SP. Cannabis use and mania symptoms: a systematic review and meta-analysis. J Affect Disord. 2015;171:39-47. PubMed PMID: 25285897.

430. van Laar M, van Dorsselaer S, Monshouwer K, de Graaf R. Does cannabis use predict the first incidence of mood and anxiety disorders in the adult population? Addiction. 2007;102(8):1251-60. PubMed PMID: 17624975.

431. Mammen G, Rueda S, Roerecke M, Bonato S, Lev-Ran S, Rehm J. Association of Cannabis With Long-Term Clinical Symptoms in Anxiety and Mood Disorders: A Systematic Review of Prospective Studies. J Clin Psychiatry. 2018;79(4). PubMed PMID: 29877641.

Chapter 8: Pregnancy, Neonatal Issues, and Childhood: Refs. 432-504

Pregnancy and Neonatal Development; The Effects of Prenatal use of Cannabis on Childhood and Adolescence Health; Cannabis Dispensaries are at odds with Health Experts Advice to Pregnant Women; The Lead Toxicity experience versus the Marijuana experience; Unintentional Cannabis ingestion in Young Children

432. Jaques SC, Kingsbury A, Henshcke P, Chomchai C, Clews S, Falconer J, et al. Cannabis, the pregnant woman and her child: weeding out the myths. J Perinatol. 2014;34(6):417-24. PubMed PMID: 24457255.

433. Burns L, Mattick RP, Cooke M. The use of record linkage to examine illicit drug use in pregnancy. Addiction. 2006;101(6):873-82. PubMed PMID: 16696631.

434. Davis E, Lee T, Weber JT, Bugden S. Cannabis use in pregnancy and breastfeeding: The pharmacist's role. Can Pharm J (Ott). 2020;153(2):95-100. PubMed PMID: 32206154; PubMed Central PMCID: 7079319. FREE

435. Baker T, Datta P, Rewers-Felkins K, Thompson H, Kallem RR, Hale TW. Transfer of Inhaled Cannabis Into Human Breast Milk. Obstet Gynecol. 2018;131(5):783-8. PubMed PMID: 29630019.

436. Dickson B, Mansfield C, Guiahi M, Allshouse AA, Borgelt LM, Sheeder J, et al. Recommendations From Cannabis Dispensaries About First-Trimester Cannabis Use. Obstet Gynecol. 2018;131(6):1031-8. PubMed PMID: 29742676; PubMed Central PMCID: 5970054. FREE

437. Agrawal A, Rogers CE, Lessov-Schlaggar CN, Carter EB, Lenze SN, Grucza RA. Alcohol, Cigarette, and Cannabis Use Between 2002 and 2016 in Pregnant Women From a Nationally Representative Sample. JAMA Pediatr. 2019;173(1):95-6. PubMed PMID: 30398527; PubMed Central PMCID: 6500767. FREE

438. Skelton KR, Hecht AA, Benjamin-Neelon SE. Recreational Cannabis Legalization in the US and Maternal Use during the Preconception, Prenatal, and

Postpartum Periods. Int J Environ Res Public Health. 2020;17(3). PubMed PMID: 32024173; PubMed Central PMCID: 7037220. FREE

439. Committee on Obstetric P. Committee Opinion No. 722: Marijuana Use During Pregnancy and Lactation. Obstet Gynecol. 2017;130(4):e205-e9. PubMed PMID: 28937574.

440. Newnam KM. The Upward Trend of Marijuana Use among Pregnant Females. Adv Neonatal Care. 2018. PubMed PMID: 29933340.

441. Volpe JJ. Commentary – Marijuana use during pregnancy and premature birth: A problem likely to worsen. J Neonatal Perinatal Med. 2020. PubMed PMID: 32007963.

442. Grant KS, Petroff R, Isoherranen N, Stella N, Burbacher TM. Cannabis use during pregnancy: Pharmacokinetics and effects on child development. Pharmacol Ther. 2018;182:133-51. PubMed PMID: 28847562; PubMed Central PMCID: 6211194. FREE

443. Massey SH, Mroczek DK, Reiss D, Miller ES, Jakubowski JA, Graham EK, et al. Additive drug-specific and sex-specific risks associated with co-use of marijuana and tobacco during pregnancy: Evidence from 3 recent developmental cohorts (2003-2015). Neurotoxicol Teratol. 2018;68:97-106. PubMed PMID: 29886244; PubMed Central PMCID: 6116514. FREE

444. Petrangelo A, Czuzoj-Shulman N, Balayla J, Abenhaim HA. Cannabis Abuse or Dependence During Pregnancy: A Population-Based Cohort Study on 12 Million Births. J Obstet Gynaecol Can. 2019;41(5):623-30. PubMed PMID: 30448107.

445. Pinky PD, Bloemer J, Smith WD, Moore T, Hong H, Suppiramaniam V, et al. Prenatal cannabinoid exposure and altered neurotransmission. Neuropharmacology. 2019;149:181-94. PubMed PMID: 30771373.

446. Sharapova SR, Phillips E, Sirocco K, Kaminski JW, Leeb RT, Rolle I. Effects of prenatal marijuana exposure on neuropsychological outcomes in children aged 1-11 years: A systematic review. Paediatr Perinat Epidemiol. 2018;32(6):512-32. PubMed PMID: 30335203; PubMed Central PMCID: 6261687. FREE

447. Scheyer A. Prenatal Exposure to Cannabis Affects the Developing Brain_The Scientist The Scientist2018. Available from: https://www.the-scientist. com/features/prenatal-exposure-to-cannabis-affects-the-developing-brain-65230.

448. Luke S, Hutcheon J, Kendall T. Cannabis Use in Pregnancy in British Columbia and Selected Birth Outcomes. J Obstet Gynaecol Can. 2019;41(9):1311-7. PubMed PMID: 30744979.

449. Howard DS, Dhanraj DN, Devaiah CG, Lambers DS. Cannabis Use Based on Urine Drug Screens in Pregnancy and Its Association With Infant Birth Weight. J Addict Med. 2019;13(6):436-41. PubMed PMID: 30908346.

450. Kharbanda EO, Vazquez-Benitez G, Kunin-Batson A, Nordin JD, Olsen A, Romitti PA. Birth and early developmental screening outcomes associated with cannabis exposure during pregnancy. J Perinatol. 2020. PubMed PMID: 31911642.

451. Crume TL, Juhl AL, Brooks-Russell A, Hall KE, Wymore E, Borgelt LM. Cannabis Use During the Perinatal Period in a State With Legalized Recreational and

Medical Marijuana: The Association Between Maternal Characteristics, Breastfeeding Patterns, and Neonatal Outcomes. J Pediatr. 2018;197:90-6. PubMed PMID: 29605394.

452. Gunn JK, Rosales CB, Center KE, Nunez A, Gibson SJ, Christ C, et al. Prenatal exposure to cannabis and maternal and child health outcomes: a systematic review and meta-analysis. BMJ Open. 2016;6(4):e009986. PubMed PMID: 27048634; PubMed Central PMCID: 4823436. FREE

453. Dekker GA, Lee SY, North RA, McCowan LM, Simpson NA, Roberts CT. Risk factors for preterm birth in an international prospective cohort of nulliparous women. PLoS One. 2012;7(7):e39154. PubMed PMID: 22815699; PubMed Central PMCID: 3398037. FREE

454. Prunet C, Delnord M, Saurel-Cubizolles MJ, Goffinet F, Blondel B. Risk factors of preterm birth in France in 2010 and changes since 1995: Results from the French National Perinatal Surveys. J Gynecol Obstet Hum Reprod. 2017;46(1):19-28. PubMed PMID: 28403953.

455. Leemaqz SY, Dekker GA, McCowan LM, Kenny LC, Myers JE, Simpson NA, et al. Maternal marijuana use has independent effects on risk for spontaneous preterm birth but not other common late pregnancy complications. Reprod Toxicol. 2016;62:77-86. PubMed PMID: 27142189.

456. Coleman-Cowger VH, Oga EA, Peters EN, Mark K. Prevalence and associated birth outcomes of co-use of Cannabis and tobacco cigarettes during pregnancy. Neurotoxicol Teratol. 2018;68:84-90. PubMed PMID: 29883744; PubMed Central PMCID: 6054553. FREE

457. Straub HL, Mou J, Drennan KJ, Pflugeisen BM. Maternal Marijuana Exposure and Birth Weight: An Observational Study Surrounding Recreational Marijuana Legalization. Am J Perinatol. 2019. PubMed PMID: 31430821.

458. Corsi DJ, Walsh L, Weiss D, Hsu H, El-Chaar D, Hawken S, et al. Association Between Self-reported Prenatal Cannabis Use and Maternal, Perinatal, and Neonatal Outcomes. JAMA. 2019;322(2):145-52. PubMed PMID: 31211826; PubMed Central PMCID: 6582262. FREE

459. Astley SJ, Little RE. Maternal marijuana use during lactation and infant development at one year. Neurotoxicol Teratol. 1990;12(2):161-8. PubMed PMID: 2333069.

460. Tennes K, Avitable N, Blackard C, Boyles C, Hassoun B, Holmes L, et al. Marijuana: prenatal and postnatal exposure in the human. NIDA Res Monogr. 1985;59:48-60. PubMed PMID: 3929132.

461. El Marroun H, Tiemeier H, Steegers EA, Jaddoe VW, Hofman A, Verhulst FC, et al. Intrauterine cannabis exposure affects fetal growth trajectories: the Generation R Study. J Am Acad Child Adolesc Psychiatry. 2009;48(12):1173-81. PubMed PMID: 19858757.

462. Corsi DJ, Donelle J, Sucha E, Hawken S, Hsu H, El-Chaar D, et al. Maternal cannabis use in pregnancy and child neurodevelopmental outcomes. Nat Med. 2020. PubMed PMID: 32778828.

462b. El Marroun H., Hudziak J.J, Tiemeier H., Creemers H., Steegers E.A.P., Jaddoe V.W.V., Hofman A., Verhulst F.C, van den Brink W., Huizink A.C. Intrauterine cannabis exposure leads to more aggressive behavior and attention problems in 18-month-old girls. Drug Alcohol

Depend .2011 Nov 1;118(2-3):470-4. PubMed
PMID_21470799 FREE

462c. Goldschmidt L., Richardson G.A., Willford J., Day
N.L.Prenatal marijuana exposure and intelligence
test performance at age 6. J Am Acad Child Adolesc
Psychiatry.2008 Mar;47(3):254-263. PubMed
PMID_18216735

463. Goldschmidt L, Day NL, Richardson GA. Effects
of prenatal marijuana exposure on child behavior
problems at age 10. Neurotoxicol Teratol. 2000;22(3):325-
36. PubMed PMID: 10840176.

464. Fried PA, Watkinson B. 12- and 24-month
neurobehavioural follow-up of children prenatally
exposed to marihuana, cigarettes and alcohol.
Neurotoxicol Teratol. 1988;10(4):305-13. PubMed
PMID: 3226373.

465. Day NL, Leech SL, Goldschmidt L. The effects of
prenatal marijuana exposure on delinquent behaviors
are mediated by measures of neurocognitive
functioning. Neurotoxicol Teratol. 2011;33(1):129-36.
PubMed PMID: 21256427; PubMed Central PMCID:
3052937. FREE

466. Guille C, Aujla R. Developmental Consequences of
Prenatal Substance Use in Children and Adolescents.
J Child Adolesc Psychopharmacol. 2019;29(7):479-86.
PubMed PMID: 31038354.

467. Gray KA, Day NL, Leech S, Richardson GA. Prenatal
marijuana exposure: effect on child depressive
symptoms at ten years of age. Neurotoxicol Teratol.
2005;27(3):439-48. PubMed PMID: 15869861.

468. Morie, K.P., Crowley, M.J., Mayes, L.C., Potenza, M.N. Prenatal drug exposure from infancy through emerging adulthood: Results from neuroimaging. Drug Alcohol Depend. 2019 May 1;198:39-53. PubMed PMID30878766 PubMed Central PMC6688747 FREE

469. Berard A. The importance of generating more data on cannabis use in pregnancy. Nat Med. 2020. PubMed PMID: 32968236.

470. Natale BV, Gustin KN, Lee K, Holloway AC, Laviolette SR, Natale DRC, et al. Delta9-tetrahydrocannabinol exposure during rat pregnancy leads to symmetrical fetal growth restriction and labyrinth-specific vascular defects in the placenta. Sci Rep. 2020;10(1):544. E PubMed PMID: 31953475; PubMed Central PMCID: 6969028. FREE

471. Breit KR, Zamudio B, Thomas JD. Altered motor development following late gestational alcohol and cannabinoid exposure in rats. Neurotoxicol Teratol. 2019;73:31-41. PubMed PMID: 30943441; PubMed Central PMCID: 6511467. FREE

472 Antonelli T, Tomasini MC, Tattoli M, Cassano T, Tanganelli S, Finetti S, et al. Prenatal exposure to the CB1 receptor agonist WIN 55,212-2 causes learning disruption associated with impaired cortical NMDA receptor function and emotional reactivity changes in rat offspring. Cereb Cortex. 2005;15(12):2013-20. PubMed PMID: 15788701.

473. Campolongo P, Trezza V, Ratano P, Palmery M, Cuomo V. Developmental consequences of perinatal cannabis exposure: behavioral and neuroendocrine effects in adult rodents. Psychopharmacology (Berl). 2011;214(1):5-15. PubMed PMID: 20556598; PubMed Central PMCID: 3045519. FREE

474. Navarro M, de Miguel R, Rodriguez de Fonseca F, Ramos JA, Fernandez-Ruiz JJ. Perinatal cannabinoid exposure modifies the sociosexual approach behavior and the mesolimbic dopaminergic activity of adult male rats. Behav Brain Res. 1996;75(1-2):91-8. PubMed PMID: 8800663.

475. Newsom RJ, Kelly SJ. Perinatal delta-9-tetrahydrocannabinol exposure disrupts social and open field behavior in adult male rats. Neurotoxicol Teratol. 2008;30(3):213-9. PubMed PMID: 18272327; PubMed Central PMCID: 2497338. FREE

476. Weimar HV, Wright HR, Warrick CR, Brown AM, Lugo JM, Freels TG, et al. Long-term effects of maternal cannabis vapor exposure on emotional reactivity, social behavior, and behavioral flexibility in offspring. Neuropharmacology. 2020:108288. PubMed PMID: 32860776.

477. Frau R, Miczan V, Traccis F, Aroni S, Pongor CI, Saba P, et al. Prenatal THC exposure produces a hyperdopaminergic phenotype rescued by pregnenolone. Nat Neurosci. 2019;22(12):1975-85. PubMed PMID: 31611707; PubMed Central PMCID: 6884689. FREE

478. del Arco I, Munoz R, Rodriguez De Fonseca F, Escudero L, Martin-Calderon JL, Navarro M, et al. Maternal exposure to the synthetic cannabinoid HU-210: effects on the endocrine and immune systems of the adult male offspring. Neuroimmunomodulation. 2000;7(1):16-26. PubMed PMID: 10601815.

479. Gillies R, Lee K, Vanin S, Laviolette SR, Holloway AC, Arany E, et al. Maternal exposure to Delta9-tetrahydrocannabinol impairs female offspring

glucose homeostasis and endocrine pancreatic development in the rat. Reprod Toxicol. 2020. PubMed PMID: 32325173.

480. Navarro M, Rodriguez de Fonseca F, Hernandez ML, Ramos JA, Fernandez-Ruiz JJ. Motor behavior and nigrostriatal dopaminergic activity in adult rats perinatally exposed to cannabinoids. Pharmacol Biochem Behav. 1994;47(1):47-58. PubMed PMID: 7906890.

481. Trezza V, Campolongo P, Cassano T, Macheda T, Dipasquale P, Carratu MR, et al. Effects of perinatal exposure to delta-9-tetrahydrocannabinol on the emotional reactivity of the offspring: a longitudinal behavioral study in Wistar rats. Psychopharmacology (Berl). 2008;198(4):529-37. PubMed PMID: 18452035.

482. Campolongo P, Trezza V, Cassano T, Gaetani S, Morgese MG, Ubaldi M, et al. Perinatal exposure to delta-9-tetrahydrocannabinol causes enduring cognitive deficits associated with alteration of cortical gene expression and neurotransmission in rats. Addict Biol. 2007;12(3-4):485-95. PubMed PMID: 17578508

483. de Salas-Quiroga A, Garcia-Rincon D, Gomez-Dominguez D, Valero M, Simon-Sanchez S, Paraiso-Luna J, et al. Long-term hippocampal interneuronopathy drives sex-dimorphic spatial memory impairment induced by prenatal THC exposure. Neuropsychopharmacology. 2020;45(5):877-86. PubMed PMID: 31982904; PubMed Central PMCID: 7075920. FREE

484. Manduca A, Servadio M, Melancia F, Schiavi S, Manzoni OJ, Trezza V. Sex-specific behavioural deficits induced at early life by prenatal exposure to the cannabinoid receptor agonist WIN55, 212-2 depend on mGlu5

receptor signalling. Br J Pharmacol. 2020;177(2):449-63. PubMed PMID: 31658362; PubMed Central PMCID: 6989958. FREE

485. Bara A, Manduca A, Bernabeu A, Borsoi M, Serviado M, Lassalle O, et al. Sex-dependent effects of in utero cannabinoid exposure on cortical function. Elife. 2018;7. PubMed PMID: 30201092; PubMed Central PMCID: 6162091. FREE

486. Ko JY, Farr SL, Tong VT, Creanga AA, Callaghan WM. Prevalence and patterns of marijuana use among pregnant and nonpregnant women of reproductive age. Am J Obstet Gynecol. 2015;213(2):201 e1- e10. PubMed PMID: 25772211.

487. Volkow ND, Han B, Compton WM, Blanco C. Marijuana Use During Stages of Pregnancy in the United States. Ann Intern Med. 2017;166(10):763-4. PubMed PMID: 28418460.

488. Volkow ND, Han B, Compton WM, McCance-Katz EF. Self-reported Medical and Nonmedical Cannabis Use Among Pregnant Women in the United States. JAMA. 2019;322(2):167-9. PubMed PMID: 31211824; PubMed Central PMCID: 6582258. FREE

489. Taylor CM, Golding J, Emond AM. Adverse effects of maternal lead levels on birth outcomes in the ALSPAC study: a prospective birth cohort study. BJOG. 2015;122(3):322-8. PubMed PMID: 24824048; PubMed Central PMCID: 4322474. FREE

490. Reuben A, Caspi A, Belsky DW, Broadbent J, Harrington H, Sugden K, et al. Association of Childhood Blood Lead Levels With Cognitive Function and Socioeconomic Status at Age 38 Years and With IQ Change and Socioeconomic Mobility Between

Childhood and Adulthood. JAMA. 2017;317(12):1244-51. PubMed PMID: 28350927; PubMed Central PMCID: 5490376. FREE

491. Zhao ZH, Zheng G, Wang T, Du KJ, Han X, Luo WJ, et al. Low-level Gestational Lead Exposure Alters Dendritic Spine Plasticity in the Hippocampus and Reduces Learning and Memory in Rats. Sci Rep. 2018;8(1):3533. PubMed PMID: 29476096; PubMed Central PMCID: 5824819. FREE

492. Lead-American Academy of Pediatrics [8/15/2020]. Available from: https://www.aap.org/en-us/advocacy-and-policy/aap-health-initiatives/lead-exposure/Pages/Lead-Exposure-in-Children.aspx.

493. Council On Environmental H. Prevention of Childhood Lead Toxicity. Pediatrics. 2016;138(1). PubMed PMID: 27325637.

494. CDC-Blood Lead Levels in Children [8/15/2020]. Available from: https://www.cdc.gov/nceh/lead/prevention/blood-lead-levels.htm?CDC_AA_refVal=https%3A%2F%2Fwww.cdc.gov%2Fnceh%2Flead%2Facclpp%2Fblood_lead_levels.htm.

495. Silva L, Zhao N, Popp S, Dow-Edwards D. Prenatal tetrahydrocannabinol (THC) alters cognitive function and amphetamine response from weaning to adulthood in the rat. Neurotoxicol Teratol. 2012;34(1):63-71. PubMed PMID: 22080840; PubMed Central PMCID: 3268847. FREE

496. CDC guidelines-Marijuana -Pregnancy [8/16/2020]. Available from: https://www.cdc.gov/marijuana/pdf/marijuana-pregnancy-508.pdf.

497. CDC-What You Need to Know About Marijuana Use and Pregnancy [8/16/2020]. Available from: https://www.cdc.gov/marijuana/factsheets/pregnancy.htm.

498. American College of Obstetricians and Gynecologists. Marijuana Use During Pregnancy and Lactation. [8/16/2020]. Available from: https://www.acog.org/clinical/clinical-guidance/committee-opinion/articles/2017/10/marijuana-use-during-pregnancy-and-lactation.

499. Richards JR, Smith NE, Moulin AK. Unintentional Cannabis Ingestion in Children: A Systematic Review. J Pediatr. 2017;190:142-52. PubMed PMID: 28888560.

500. Carvalho A, Evans-Gilbert T. The Pathophysiology of Marijuana-induced Encephalopathy and Possible Epilepsy after Ingestion in Children: A Case Series. Innov Clin Neurosci. 2019;16(3-4):16-8. PubMed PMID: 31214478; PubMed Central PMCID: 6538397. FREE

501. Wong KU, Baum CR. Acute Cannabis Toxicity. Pediatr Emerg Care. 2019;35(11):799-804. PubMed PMID: 31688799.

502. Wang GS, Banerji S, Contreras AE, Hall KE. Marijuana exposures in Colorado, reported to regional poison centre, 2000-2018. Inj Prev. 2020;26(2):184-6. PubMed PMID: 31676510.

503. Claudet I, Mouvier S, Labadie M, Manin C, Michard-Lenoir AP, Eyer D, et al. Unintentional Cannabis Intoxication in Toddlers. Pediatrics. 2017;140(3). PubMed PMID: 28808073.

504. Claudet I, Le Breton M, Brehin C, Franchitto N. A 10-year review of cannabis exposure in children under

3-years of age: do we need a more global approach? Eur J Pediatr. 2017;176(4):553-6. PubMed PMID: 28210835.

Chapter 9: Other Very Important Heath-related Stuff: Refs. 505-572

Your Heart and blood vessels; Stroke; Transient Ischemic Attacks; Sleep; Testicular Cancer; Cannabinoid Hyperemesis Syndrome

505. Hiley CR. Endocannabinoids and the heart. J Cardiovasc Pharmacol. 2009;53(4):267-76.. PubMed PMID: 19276990; PubMed Central PMCID: 2728560. FREE

506. Richter JS, Quenardelle V, Rouyer O, Raul JS, Beaujeux R, Geny B, et al. A Systematic Review of the Complex Effects of Cannabinoids on Cerebral and Peripheral Circulation in Animal Models. Front Physiol. 2018;9:622. PubMed PMID: 29896112; PubMed Central PMCID: 5986896. FREE

507. Richards JR, Blohm E, Toles KA, Jarman AF, Ely DF, Elder JW. The association of cannabis use and cardiac dysrhythmias: a systematic review. Clin Toxicol (Phila). 2020:1-9. 7. PubMed PMID: 32267189.

508. Richards JR, Bing ML, Moulin AK, Elder JW, Rominski RT, Summers PJ, et al. Cannabis use and acute coronary syndrome. Clin Toxicol (Phila). 2019;57(10):831-41. PubMed PMID: 30964363.

509. Lodhi MU, Singh S, Ruiz Mercedes B, Malik FA, Desai R. Concerning trends in cardiogenic shock-related admissions among United States cannabis users. Int J Cardiol Heart Vasc. 2020;30:100614. PubMed PMID: 32817882; PubMed Central PMCID: 7424209. FREE

510. Desai R, Patel U, Deshmukh A, Sachdeva R, Kumar G. Burden of arrhythmia in recreational marijuana users. Int J Cardiol. 2018;264:91-2. PubMed PMID: 29642998.

511. Desai R, Patel U, Sharma S, Amin P, Bhuva R, Patel MS, et al. Recreational Marijuana Use and Acute Myocardial Infarction: Insights from Nationwide Inpatient Sample in the United States. Cureus. 2017;9(11):e1816. PubMed PMID: 29312837; PubMed Central PMCID: 5752226. FREE

512. Ramphul K, Mejias SG, Joynauth J. Cocaine, Amphetamine, and Cannabis Use Increases the Risk of Acute Myocardial Infarction in Teenagers. Am J Cardiol. 2019;123(2):354. PubMed PMID: 30477798.

513. Mittleman MA, Lewis RA, Maclure M, Sherwood JB, Muller JE. Triggering myocardial infarction by marijuana. Circulation. 2001;103(23):2805-9. PubMed PMID: 11401936.

514. Pacher P, Steffens S, Hasko G, Schindler TH, Kunos G. Cardiovascular effects of marijuana and synthetic cannabinoids: the good, the bad, and the ugly. Nat Rev Cardiol. 2018;15(3):151-66. PubMed PMID: 28905873.

515. Chaphekar A, Campbell M, Middleman AB. With a High, Comes a Low: A Case of Heavy Marijuana Use and Bradycardia in an Adolescent. Clin Pediatr (Phila). 2019;58(14):1550-3. PubMed PMID: 31179732.

516. Patel RS, Manocha P, Patel J, Patel R, Tankersley WE. Cannabis Use Is an Independent Predictor for Acute Myocardial Infarction Related Hospitalization in Younger Population. J Adolesc Health. 2019. PubMed PMID: 31611137.

517. Parekh T, Pemmasani S, Desai R. Marijuana Use Among Young Adults (18-44 Years of Age) and Risk of Stroke: A Behavioral Risk Factor Surveillance System Survey Analysis. Stroke. 2019:STROKEAHA119027828. PubMed PMID: 31707926.

518. Ravi D, Ghasemiesfe M, Korenstein D, Cascino T, Keyhani S. Associations Between Marijuana Use and Cardiovascular Risk Factors and Outcomes: A Systematic Review. Ann Intern Med. 2018;168(3):187-94. PubMed PMID: 29357394; PubMed Central PMCID: 6157910. FREE

519. Desai R, Shamim S, Patel K, Sadolikar A, Kaur VP, Bhivandkar S, et al. Primary Causes of Hospitalizations and Procedures, Predictors of In-hospital Mortality, and Trends in Cardiovascular and Cerebrovascular Events Among Recreational Marijuana Users: A Five-year Nationwide Inpatient Assessment in the United States. Cureus. 2018;10(8):e3195. PubMed PMID: 30402363; PubMed Central PMCID: 6200442. FREE

520. Goel A, McGuinness B, Jivraj NK, Wijeysundera DN, Mittleman MA, Bateman BT, et al. Cannabis Use Disorder and Perioperative Outcomes in Major Elective Surgeries: A Retrospective Cohort Analysis. Anesthesiology. 2019. PubMed PMID: 31789638.

521. Page RL, 2nd, Allen LA, Kloner RA, Carriker CR, Martel C, Morris AA, et al. Medical Marijuana, Recreational Cannabis, and Cardiovascular Health: A Scientific Statement From the American Heart Association. Circulation. Sep 8 2020; 142(10) PubMed PMID: 32752884.

522. Vidot DC, Powers M, Gonzalez R, Jayaweera DT, Roy S, Dong C, et al. Blood Pressure and Marijuana Use: Results from a Decade of NHANES Data. Am J Health Behav. 2019;43(5):887-97. PubMed PMID: 31439096.

523. Cardiovascular disease- Heart.org [8/25/2020]. Available from: https://www.heart.org/en/news/2019/01/31/cardiovascular-diseases-affect-nearly-half-of-american-adults-statistics-show.

524. Diabetes statistics-Diabetes.org [8/25/2020]. Available from: https://www.diabetes.org/resources/statistics/statistics-about-diabetes.

525. Jamil M, Zafar A, Adeel Faizi S, Zawar I. Stroke from Vasospasm due to Marijuana Use: Can Cannabis Synergistically with Other Medications Trigger Cerebral Vasospasm? Case Rep Neurol Med. 2016;2016:5313795. PubMed PMID: 27833768; PubMed Central PMCID: 5090067. FREE

526. Baskaran J, Anantha Narayanan M, Vakhshoorzadeh J, Ahmad A, Bertog S. Marijuana-induced Coronary Vasospasm with Persistent Inter-coronary Connection: A Case Report and Review of Literature. Cureus. 2019;11(6):e4799. PubMed PMID: 31497413; PubMed Central PMCID: 6726350. FREE

527. Jack Herer Wikipedia [12-7-2020]. Available from: https://en.wikipedia.org/wiki/Jack_Herer.

528. Arrythmia -American Heart Association. Available from: https://www.heart.org/en/health-topics/arrhythmia.

529. Ramphul K, Joynauth J. Cardiac Arrhythmias Among Teenagers Using Cannabis in the United States. Am J Cardiol. 2019;124(12):1966. PubMed PMID: 31653358.

530. Van Keer JM. Cannabis-Induced Third-Degree AV Block. Case Rep Emerg Med. 2019;2019:5037356. PubMed PMID: 31637064; PubMed Central PMCID: 6766110. FREE

531. Stroke-American Stroke Association. Available from: https://www.stroke.org/en/about-stroke.

532. Sharma D, Dahal U, Yu E. Complete Occlusion of Bilateral Internal Carotid Artery in a Marijuana Smoker: A Case Report. J Clin Med Res. 2019;11(4):305-8. PubMed PMID: 30937123; PubMed Central PMCID: 6436573. FREE

533. Desai R, Singh S, Patel K, Goyal H, Shah M, Mansuri Z, et al. Stroke in young cannabis users (18-49 years): National trends in hospitalizations and outcomes. Int J Stroke. 2019:1747493019895651. PubMed PMID: 31870242.

534. Transient Ischemic Attacks Mayo Clinic [12-7-2020]. Available from: https://www.mayoclinic.org/diseases-conditions/transient-ischemic-attack/symptoms-causes/syc-20355679.

535. Transient Ischemic Attacks www.stroke.org [12-7-2020]. Available from: https://www.stroke.org/en/about-stroke/types-of-stroke/tia-transient-ischemic-attack.

536. Hemachandra D, McKetin R, Cherbuin N, Anstey KJ. Heavy cannabis users at elevated risk of stroke: evidence from a general population survey. Aust N Z J Public Health. 2016;40(3):226-30. Epub 2015/11/13. doi: 10.1111/1753-6405.12477. PubMed PMID: 26558539. FREE

537. Mouzak A, Agathos P, Kerezoudi E, Mantas A, Vourdeli-Yiannakoura E. Transient ischemic attack in heavy cannabis smokers—how 'safe' is it? Eur Neurol. 2000;44(1):42-4. Epub 2000/07/15. doi: 10.1159/000008191. PubMed PMID: 10894994. FREE

538. Murillo-Rodriguez E, Cabeza R, Mendez-Diaz M, Navarro L, Prospero-Garcia O. Anandamide-induced sleep is blocked by SR141716A, a CB1 receptor antagonist and by U73122, a phospholipase C inhibitor. Neuroreport. 2001;12(10):2131-6. PubMed PMID: 11447321.

539. Rueda-Orozco PE, Soria-Gomez E, Montes-Rodriguez CJ, Perez-Morales M, Prospero-Garcia O. Intrahippocampal administration of anandamide increases REM sleep. Neurosci Lett. 2010;473(2):158-62. PubMed PMID: 20188142.

540. Clendinning J. Observations on the medicinal properties of the Cannabis Sativa of India. Med Chir Trans. 1843;26:188-210. PubMed PMID: 20895771; PubMed Central PMCID: 2116906. FREE

541. Gates PJ, Albertella L, Copeland J. The effects of cannabinoid administration on sleep: a systematic review of human studies. Sleep Med Rev. 2014;18(6):477-87. PubMed PMID: 24726015.

542. Babson KA, Sottile J, Morabito D. Cannabis, Cannabinoids, and Sleep: a Review of the Literature. Curr Psychiatry Rep. 2017;19(4):23. PubMed PMID: 28349316.

543. Gorelick DA, Goodwin RS, Schwilke E, Schroeder JR, Schwope DM, Kelly DL, et al. Around-the-clock oral THC effects on sleep in male chronic daily cannabis smokers. Am J Addict. 2013;22(5):510-4. PubMed PMID: 23952899; PubMed Central PMCID: 4537525. FREE

544. Campbell LM, Tang B, Watson CW, Higgins M, Cherner M, Henry BL, et al. Cannabis use is associated with greater total sleep time in middle-aged and older adults with and without HIV: A preliminary report utilizing digital health technologies. Cannabis. 2020;3(2):180-9. PubMed PMID: 32905460; PubMed Central PMCID: 7470214. FREE

545. Suraev AS, Marshall NS, Vandrey R, McCartney D, Benson MJ, McGregor IS, et al. Cannabinoid therapies in the management of sleep disorders: A systematic review of preclinical and clinical studies. Sleep Med Rev. 2020;53:101339. PubMed PMID: 32603954.

546. Carley DW, Prasad B, Reid KJ, Malkani R, Attarian H, Abbott SM, et al. Pharmacotherapy of Apnea by Cannabimimetic Enhancement, the PACE Clinical Trial: Effects of Dronabinol in Obstructive Sleep Apnea. Sleep. 2018;41(1). PubMed PMID: 29121334; PubMed Central PMCID: 5806568. FREE

547. Russo EB, Guy GW, Robson PJ. Cannabis, pain, and sleep: lessons from therapeutic clinical trials of Sativex, a cannabis-based medicine. Chem Biodivers. 2007;4(8):1729-43. PubMed PMID: 17712817.

548. Shannon S, Lewis N, Lee H, Hughes S. Cannabidiol in Anxiety and Sleep: A Large Case Series. Perm J. 2019;23:18-041. PubMed PMID: 30624194; PubMed Central PMCID: 6326553. FREE

549. Megelin T, Ghorayeb I. Cannabis for restless legs syndrome: a report of six patients. Sleep Med. 2017;36:182-3. PubMed PMID: 28655453.

550. Jetly R, Heber A, Fraser G, Boisvert D. The efficacy of nabilone, a synthetic cannabinoid, in the treatment of PTSD-associated nightmares: A preliminary

randomized, double-blind, placebo-controlled crossover design study. Psychoneuroendocrinology. 2015;51:585-8. PubMed PMID: 25467221.

551. Bolla KI, Lesage SR, Gamaldo CE, Neubauer DN, Funderburk FR, Cadet JL, et al. Sleep disturbance in heavy marijuana users. Sleep. 2008;31(6):901-8. PubMed PMID: 18548836; PubMed Central PMCID: 2442418. FREE

552. Budney AJ, Hughes JR, Moore BA, Vandrey R. Review of the validity and significance of cannabis withdrawal syndrome. Am J Psychiatry. 2004;161(11):1967-77. PubMed PMID: 15514394.

553. Angarita GA, Emadi N, Hodges S, Morgan PT. Sleep abnormalities associated with alcohol, cannabis, cocaine, and opiate use: a comprehensive review. Addict Sci Clin Pract. 2016;11(1):9. PubMed PMID: 27117064; PubMed Central PMCID: 4845302. FREE

554. Lund HG, Reider BD, Whiting AB, Prichard JR. Sleep patterns and predictors of disturbed sleep in a large population of college students. J Adolesc Health. 2010;46(2):124-32. PubMed PMID: 20113918.

555. Drazdowski TK, Kliewer WL, Marzell M. College students' using marijuana to sleep relates to frequency, problematic use, and sleep problems. J Am Coll Health. 2019:1-10. PubMed PMID: 31498749; PubMed Central PMCID: 7061072. FREE

556. Trabert B, Sigurdson AJ, Sweeney AM, Strom SS, McGlynn KA. Marijuana use and testicular germ cell tumors. Cancer. 2011;117(4):848-53. PubMed PMID: 20925043; PubMed Central PMCID: 3017734. FREE

557. Lewis SE, Maccarrone M. Endocannabinoids, sperm biology and human fertility. Pharmacol Res. 2009;60(2):126-31. PubMed PMID: 19559363.

558. du Plessis SS, Agarwal A, Syriac A. Marijuana, phytocannabinoids, the endocannabinoid system, and male fertility. J Assist Reprod Genet. 2015;32(11):1575-88. PubMed PMID: 26277482; PubMed Central PMCID: 4651943. FREE

559. Daling JR, Doody DR, Sun X, Trabert BL, Weiss NS, Chen C, et al. Association of marijuana use and the incidence of testicular germ cell tumors. Cancer. 2009;115(6):1215-23. PubMed PMID: 19204904; PubMed Central PMCID: 2759698. FREE

560. Callaghan RC, Allebeck P, Akre O, McGlynn KA, Sidorchuk A. Cannabis Use and Incidence of Testicular Cancer: A 42-Year Follow-up of Swedish Men between 1970 and 2011. Cancer Epidemiol Biomarkers Prev. 2017;26(11):1644-52. PubMed PMID: 29093004; PubMed Central PMCID: 5812006. FREE

561. Ghasemiesfe M, Barrow B, Leonard S, Keyhani S, Korenstein D. Association Between Marijuana Use and Risk of Cancer: A Systematic Review and Meta-analysis. JAMA Netw Open. 2019;2(11):e1916318. PubMed PMID: 31774524; PubMed Central PMCID: 6902836. FREE

562. Cannabinoid Hyperemesis Syndrome Wikipedia [4-21-20]. Available from: https://en.wikipedia.org/wiki/Cannabinoid_hyperemesis_syndrome.

563. Allen JH, de Moore GM, Heddle R, Twartz JC. Cannabinoid hyperemesis: cyclical hyperemesis in association with chronic cannabis abuse. Gut. 2004;53(11):1566-70. PubMed PMID: 15479672; PubMed Central PMCID: 1774264. FREE

564. Chu F, Cascella M. Cannabinoid Hyperemesis Syndrome. StatPearls. Treasure Island (FL)2020. PubMed PMID: 31751105. FREE

565. Attout H, Amichi S, Josse F, Appavoupoule V, Randriajohany A, Thirapathi Y. Cannabis Hyperemesis Syndrome: A Still Under-Recognized Syndrome. Eur J Case Rep Intern Med. 2020;7(5):001588. PubMed PMID: 32399447; PubMed Central PMCID: 7213821. FREE

566. Glauser W. Nausea-inducing illness caused by cannabis still underdiagnosed. CMAJ. 2019;191(47):E1316-E7. PubMed PMID: 31767711; PubMed Central PMCID: 6877360. FREE

567. Sontineni SP, Chaudhary S, Sontineni V, Lanspa SJ. Cannabinoid hyperemesis syndrome: clinical diagnosis of an underrecognised manifestation of chronic cannabis abuse. World J Gastroenterol. 2009;15(10):1264-6. PubMed PMID: 19291829; PubMed Central PMCID: 2658859. FREE

568. Habboushe J, Rubin A, Liu H, Hoffman RS. The Prevalence of Cannabinoid Hyperemesis Syndrome Among Regular Marijuana Smokers in an Urban Public Hospital. Basic Clin Pharmacol Toxicol. 2018;122(6):660-2. PubMed PMID: 29327809.

569. Cannabinoid Hyperemesis Syndrome Cedars-Sinai [4-21-20]. Available from: https://www.cedars-sinai.org/health-library/diseases-and-conditions/c/cannabinoid-hyperemesis-syndrome.html.

570. Nicolson SE, Denysenko L, Mulcare JL, Vito JP, Chabon B. Cannabinoid hyperemesis syndrome: a case series and review of previous reports. Psychosomatics. 2012;53(3):212-9. PubMed PMID: 22480624.

571. Lu ML, Agito MD. Cannabinoid hyperemesis syndrome: Marijuana is both antiemetic and proemetic. Cleve Clin J Med. 2015;82(7):429-34. PubMed PMID: 26185942.

572. Parekh JD, Wozniak SE, Khan K, Dutta SK. Cannabinoid hyperemesis syndrome. BMJ Case Rep. 2016;2016. PubMed PMID: 26791124; PubMed Central PMCID: 4735328. FREE

Chapter 10: Societal Related Stuff: Refs. 573-633
Educational Achievement; Motivation; Employment and Jobs; Conflating Legalization issues with Health Issues; Driving; Violence; Suicide; and PTSD

573. Linden-Carmichael AN, Kloska DD, Evans-Polce R, Lanza ST, Patrick ME. College degree attainment by age of first marijuana use and parental education. Subst Abus. 2019;40(1):66-70. PubMed PMID: 30475168; PubMed Central PMCID: 6535370. FREE

574. Fergusson DM, Horwood LJ, Beautrais AL. Cannabis and educational achievement. Addiction. 2003;98(12):1681-92. PubMed PMID: 14651500.

574b. Ryan AK. The lasting effects of marijuana use on educational attainment in midlife. Subst Use Misuse. 2010;45(4):554-97. PubMed PMID: 20141465.

575. Homel J, Thompson K, Leadbeater B. Trajectories of marijuana use in youth ages 15-25: implications for postsecondary education experiences. J Stud Alcohol Drugs. 2014;75(4):674-83. PubMed PMID: 24988266; PubMed Central PMCID: 4905757. FREE

576. Ashdown-Franks G, Sabiston CM, Vancampfort D, Smith L, Firth J, Solmi M, et al. Cannabis use and physical activity among 89,777 adolescents aged 12-15 years from

21 low- and middle-income countries. Drug Alcohol Depend. 2019;205:107584. PubMed PMID: 31707273.

577. Vancampfort D, Firth J, Smith L, Stubbs B, Rosenbaum S, Van Damme T, et al. Cannabis use and leisure-time sedentary behavior among 94,035 adolescents aged 12-15years from 24 low- and middle-income countries. Addict Behav. 2019;99:106104. PubMed PMID: 31470242.

578. Pacheco-Colon I, Limia JM, Gonzalez R. Nonacute effects of cannabis use on motivation and reward sensitivity in humans: A systematic review. Psychol Addict Behav. 2018;32(5):497-507. PubMed PMID: 29963875; PubMed Central PMCID: 6062456. FREE

579. Petrucci AS, LaFrance EM, Cuttler C. A Comprehensive Examination of the Links between Cannabis Use and Motivation. Subst Use Misuse. 2020:1-10. PubMed PMID: 32100610.

580. Silins E, Fergusson DM, Patton GC, Horwood LJ, Olsson CA, Hutchinson DM, et al. Adolescent substance use and educational attainment: An integrative data analysis comparing cannabis and alcohol from three Australasian cohorts. Drug Alcohol Depend. 2015;156:90-6. PubMed PMID: 26409754.

581. Silins E, Horwood LJ, Patton GC, Fergusson DM, Olsson CA, Hutchinson DM, et al. Young adult sequelae of adolescent cannabis use: an integrative analysis. Lancet Psychiatry. 2014;1(4):286-93. PubMed PMID: 26360862.

582. Ellickson PL, Martino SC, Collins RL. Marijuana use from adolescence to young adulthood: multiple developmental trajectories and their associated

outcomes. Health Psychol. 2004;23(3):299-307. PubMed PMID: 15099171.

583. Epstein M, Hill KG, Nevell AM, Guttmannova K, Bailey JA, Abbott RD, et al. Trajectories of marijuana use from adolescence into adulthood: Environmental and individual correlates. Dev Psychol. 2015;51(11):1650-63. PubMed PMID: 26389603; PubMed Central PMCID: 4623873. FREE

584. Popovici I, French MT. Cannabis use, employment, and income: fixed-effects analysis of panel data. J Behav Health Serv Res. 2014;41(2):185-202. PubMed PMID: 23793384; PubMed Central PMCID: 3867578. FREE

585. Okechukwu CA, Molino J, Soh Y. Associations Between Marijuana Use and Involuntary Job Loss in the United States: Representative Longitudinal and Cross-Sectional Samples. J Occup Environ Med. 2019;61(1):21-8. PubMed PMID: 30256305; PubMed Central PMCID: 6314892. FREE

586. Arria AM, Garnier-Dykstra LM, Cook ET, Caldeira KM, Vincent KB, Baron RA, et al. Drug use patterns in young adulthood and post-college employment. Drug Alcohol Depend. 2013;127(1-3):23-30. PubMed PMID: 22743161; PubMed Central PMCID: 3463732. FREE

587. DeSimone J. Illegal drug use and employment. Journal of Labor Economics. 2002;20:952-77.

588. Airagnes G, Lemogne C, Meneton P, Plessz M, Goldberg M, Hoertel N, et al. Alcohol, tobacco and cannabis use are associated with job loss at follow-up: Findings from the CONSTANCES cohort. PLoS One. 2019;14(9):e0222361. PubMed PMID: 31498849; PubMed Central PMCID: 6733456 FREE

589. Kaestner R. New estimates of the effect of marijuana and cocaine use on wages. Industrial and Labor Relations Review. 1994;47:454–70.

590. Rovai L, Maremmani AG, Pacini M, Pani PP, Rugani F, Lamanna F, et al. Negative dimension in psychiatry. Amotivational syndrome as a paradigm of negative symptoms in substance abuse. Riv Psichiatr. 2013;48(1):1-9. PubMed PMID: 23438696.

591. Movie The Big Lebowski Wikipedia. Available from: https://en.wikipedia.org/wiki/The_Big_Lebowski.

592. Big Lebowski-quotes [6-22-20]. Available from: https://uproxx.com/movies/20-big-lebowski-quotes/.

593. McGlothlin WH, West LJ. The marihuana problem: an overview. Am J Psychiatry. 1968;125(3):126-34. PubMed PMID: 5667203.

594. Lawn W, Freeman TP, Pope RA, Joye A, Harvey L, Hindocha C, et al. Acute and chronic effects of cannabinoids on effort-related decision-making and reward learning: an evaluation of the cannabis 'amotivational' hypotheses. Psychopharmacology (Berl). 2016;233(19-20):3537-52. PubMed PMID: 27585792; PubMed Central PMCID: 5021728. FREE

595. Brands B, Mann RE, Wickens CM, Sproule B, Stoduto G, Sayer GS, et al. Acute and residual effects of smoked cannabis: Impact on driving speed and lateral control, heart rate, and self-reported drug effects. Drug Alcohol Depend. 2019;205:107641. PubMed PMID: 31678833.

596. Bondallaz P, Favrat B, Chtioui H, Fornari E, Maeder P, Giroud C. Cannabis and its effects on driving skills. Forensic Sci Int. 2016;268:92-102. PubMed PMID: 27701009.

597. Eichelberger AH. Marijuana use and driving in Washington State: Risk perceptions and behaviors before and after implementation of retail sales. Traffic Inj Prev. 2019;20(1):23-9. PubMed PMID: 30822133.

598. Doroudgar S, Mae Chuang H, Bohnert K, Canedo J, Burrowes S, Perry PJ. Effects of chronic marijuana use on driving performance. Traffic Inj Prev. 2018;19(7):680-6. PubMed PMID: 30411981.

599. Cook AC, Leung G, Smith RA. Marijuana Decriminalization, Medical Marijuana Laws, and Fatal Traffic Crashes in US Cities, 2010-2017. Am J Public Health. 2020;110(3):363-9. PubMed PMID: 31944840.

600. Baldock M, Lindsay T. Illicit drugs are now more common than alcohol among South Australian crash-involved drivers and riders. Traffic Inj Prev. 2020;21(1):1-6. E PubMed PMID: 31999482.

601. Nazif-Munoz JI, Oulhote Y, Ouimet MC. The association between legalisation of cannabis use and traffic deaths in Uruguay. Addiction. 2020. PubMed PMID: 32003494.

602. Sukhawathanakul P, Thompson K, Brubacher J, Leadbeater B. Marijuana trajectories and associations with driving risk behaviors in Canadian youth. Traffic Inj Prev. 2019;20(5):472-7. PubMed PMID: 31194581.

603. Asbridge M, Hayden JA, Cartwright JL. Acute cannabis consumption and motor vehicle collision risk: systematic review of observational studies and meta-analysis. BMJ. 2012;344:e536. PubMed PMID: 22323502; PubMed Central PMCID: 3277079. FREE

604. Miller NS, Ipeku R, Oberbarnscheidt T. A Review of Cases of Marijuana and Violence. Int J Environ Res Public Health. 2020;17(5). PubMed PMID: 32121373.

605. Dugre JR, Dellazizzo L, Giguere CE, Potvin S, Dumais A. Persistency of Cannabis Use Predicts Violence following Acute Psychiatric Discharge. Front Psychiatry. 2017;8:176. PubMed PMID: 28983261; PubMed Central PMCID: 5613094. FREE

606. Arseneault L, Moffitt TE, Caspi A, Taylor PJ, Silva PA. Mental disorders and violence in a total birth cohort: results from the Dunedin Study. Arch Gen Psychiatry. 2000;57(10):979-86. PubMed PMID: 11015816.

607. Beaudoin M, Potvin S, Giguere CE, Discepola SL, Dumais A. Persistent cannabis use as an independent risk factor for violent behaviors in patients with schizophrenia. NPJ Schizophr. 2020;6(1):14. PubMed PMID: 32393793.

608. Norstrom T, Rossow I. Cannabis use and violence: Is there a link? Scand J Public Health. 2014;42(4):358-63. PubMed PMID: 24608093.

609. Kylie Lee KS, Sukavatvibul K, Conigrave KM. Cannabis use and violence in three remote Aboriginal Australian communities: Analysis of clinic presentations. Transcult Psychiatry. 2015;52(6):827-39. PubMed PMID: 26045571.

610. Rao H, Luty J, Trathen B. Characteristics of patients who are violent to staff and towards other people from a community mental health service in South East England. J Psychiatr Ment Health Nurs. 2007;14(8):753-7. PubMed PMID: 18039298.

611. Moulin V, Baumann P, Gholamrezaee M, Alameda L, Palix J, Gasser J, et al. Cannabis, a Significant Risk Factor for Violent Behavior in the Early Phase Psychosis. Two Patterns of Interaction of Factors Increase the Risk of Violent Behavior: Cannabis Use Disorder and Impulsivity; Cannabis Use Disorder, Lack of Insight and

Treatment Adherence. Front Psychiatry. 2018;9:294. PubMed PMID: 30022956; PubMed Central PMCID: 6039574. FREE

612. Rolin SA, Marino LA, Pope LG, Compton MT, Lee RJ, Rosenfeld B, et al. Recent violence and legal involvement among young adults with early psychosis enrolled in Coordinated Specialty Care. Early Interv Psychiatry. 2019;13(4):832-40. PubMed PMID: 29740953; PubMed Central PMCID: 6226380. FREE

613. Krakowski MI, De Sanctis P, Foxe JJ, Hoptman MJ, Nolan K, Kamiel S, et al. Disturbances in Response Inhibition and Emotional Processing as Potential Pathways to Violence in Schizophrenia: A High-Density Event-Related Potential Study. Schizophr Bull. 2016;42(4):963-74. PubMed PMID: 26895845; PubMed Central PMCID: 4903062. FREE

614. Berenson A. Tell Your Children- The Truth About Marijuana, Mental Illness and Violence.: Free Press; 2019.

615. Berenson A. Marijuana, Mental illness, and Violence. Mo Med. 2019;116(6):446-9. PubMed PMID: 31911714; PubMed Central PMCID: 6913867. FREE

616. Johnson RM, LaValley M, Schneider KE, Musci RJ, Pettoruto K, Rothman EF. Marijuana use and physical dating violence among adolescents and emerging adults: A systematic review and meta-analysis. Drug Alcohol Depend. 2017;174:47-57. PubMed PMID: 28314193; PubMed Central PMCID: 5521998. FREE

617. Shorey RC, Haynes E, Brem M, Florimbio AR, Grigorian H, Stuart GL. Marijuana use is associated with intimate partner violence perpetration among men arrested for domestic violence. Transl Issues Psychol Sci.

2018;4(1):108-18. PubMed PMID: 30829345; PubMed Central PMCID: 5663469. FREE

618. Suicide ideation Wikipedia. Available from: https://en.wikipedia.org/wiki/Suicidal_ideation.

619. NIMH Suicide. Available from: https://www.nimh.nih.gov/health/publications/suicide-faq/index.shtml.

621. Sellers CM, Diaz-Valdes Iriarte A, Wyman Battalen A, O'Brien KHM. Alcohol and marijuana use as daily predictors of suicide ideation and attempts among adolescents prior to psychiatric hospitalization. Psychiatry Res. 2019;273:672-7. PubMed PMID: 31207851.

622. Halladay JE, Munn C, Boyle M, Jack SM, Georgiades K. Temporal Changes in the Cross-Sectional Associations between Cannabis Use, Suicidal Ideation, and Depression in a Nationally Representative Sample of Canadian Adults in 2012 Compared to 2002. Can J Psychiatry. 2020;65(2):115-23. PubMed PMID: 31177831; PubMed Central PMCID: 6997972. FREE

623. Carvalho AF, Stubbs B, Vancampfort D, Kloiber S, Maes M, Firth J, et al. Cannabis use and suicide attempts among 86,254 adolescents aged 12-15 years from 21 low- and middle-income countries. Eur Psychiatry. 2019;56:8-13. PubMed PMID: 30447436.

624. Borges G, Bagge CL, Orozco R. A literature review and meta-analyses of cannabis use and suicidality. J Affect Disord. 2016;195:63-74. PubMed PMID: 26872332.

625. Tom Forcade. Available from: https://en.wikipedia.org/wiki/Tom_Forcade.

626. Tom Forcade-High
Times. Available from: https://hightimes.com/culture/
high-times-greats-life-high-times-tom-forcade/.

627. Lake S, Kerr T, Buxton J, Walsh Z, Marshall BD, Wood
E, et al. Does cannabis use modify the effect of post-
traumatic stress disorder on severe depression and
suicidal ideation? Evidence from a population-based
cross-sectional study of Canadians. J Psychopharmacol.
2020;34(2):181-8. PubMed PMID: 31684805.

628. Hindocha C, Cousijn J, Rall M, Bloomfield MAP. The
Effectiveness of Cannabinoids in the Treatment of
Posttraumatic Stress Disorder (PTSD): A Systematic
Review. J Dual Diagn. 2020;16(1):120-39. PubMed PMID:
31479625.

629. Allan NP, Ashrafioun L, Kolnogorova K, Raines AM,
Hoge CW, Stecker T. Interactive effects of PTSD and
substance use on suicidal ideation and behavior in
military personnel: Increased risk from marijuana use.
Depress Anxiety. 2019;36(11):1072-9. PubMed PMID:
31475423.

630. Bilevicius E, Sommer JL, Asmundson GJG, El-Gabalawy
R. Associations of PTSD, chronic pain, and their
comorbidity on cannabis use disorder: Results
from an American nationally representative study.
Depress Anxiety. 2019;36(11):1036-46. PubMed PMID:
31356731.

631. Wilkinson ST, Stefanovics E, Rosenheck RA.
Marijuana use is associated with worse outcomes in
symptom severity and violent behavior in patients
with posttraumatic stress disorder. J Clin Psychiatry.
2015;76(9):1174-80. PubMed PMID: 26455669; PubMed
Central PMCID: 6258013. FREE

632. Yeh CL, Levar N, Broos HC, Dechert A, Potter K, Eden EA, et al. White matter integrity differences associated with post-traumatic stress disorder are not normalized by concurrent marijuana use. Psychiatry Res Neuroimaging. 2020;295:111017. PubMed PMID: 31760337.

633. Adkisson K, Cunningham KC, Dedert EA, Dennis MF, Calhoun PS, Elbogen EB, et al. Cannabis Use Disorder and Post-Deployment Suicide Attempts in Iraq/Afghanistan-Era Veterans. Arch Suicide Res. 2019;23(4):678-87. PubMed PMID: 29952737; PubMed Central PMCID: 6525085. FREE